"The great challenge in pastoral ministry today is for the minister to integrate a sound foundational theology into pastoral activity. *Growing Through Pain and Suffering* is a significant step in this process of integration because van der Poel connects the human experience of suffering with the best of the theological tradition. I recommend this work to all pastoral ministers who search with others for meaning in the context of pain."

Edward van Merrienboer, O.P., D.Min.
Chair, Dept. of Theology & Philosophy
Barry University, Miami Shores, Florida

"Befriending suffering through understanding and courage is at the core of this opportune book. Rev. van der Poel has brought much experience and penetrating insights to the mysterious experience of suffering. People involved in pastoral care at all levels will benefit greatly from this fine text."

Robert F. Morneau
Auxiliary Bishop of Green Bay

"This book is addressed to all who have to deal with pain and suffering. It does not indulge in pious platitudes nor pretend to have easy answers to all questions. It does emphasize that the life situation and the attitude toward suffering of those in pain are the starting point for those who wish to minister to them.

"Father van der Poel is well qualified for the task he has set himself. For many years he has alternated between times of actual pastoral care and times for study and reflection on the theology and psychology of pastoral care. His many books and articles reflect this methodology, and this book is no exception. It deserves wide distribution. It will be a great service to those who suffer and to those who minister to them."

Christopher P. Promis, C.S.Sp.
Provincial Superior

GROWING THROUGH

Cornelius J. van der Poel

XXIII
TWENTY-THIRD PUBLICATIONS
Mystic, Connecticut 06355

1. Spiritual journey - suffering
2. Spiritual life
3. Pain - Religious aspects

Twenty-Third Publications
185 Willow Street
P.O. Box 180
Mystic, CT 06355
(203) 536-2611
800-321-0411

© Copyright 1995 Cornelius J. van der Poel. All rights reserved. No part of this publication may be reproduced in any manner without prior written permission of the publisher. Write to Permissions Editor.

ISBN 0-89622-636-0
Library of Congress Catalog Card Number 94-61812
Printed in the U.S.A.

NA-1394

Preface

Everyone who opens this book has had personal experiences of pain and suffering, or at least has seen pain and suffering in others. Through modern technology we are eyewitnesses to gruesome slaughters, deadly famine, disastrous accidents, and natural disasters. The frightening disease of AIDS in its various degrees and forms brings us pictures of emaciated victims who often cling to life and add to the frustrations of physicians and other caregivers. We may also know someone considering physician-assisted suicide, and wonder what we can say to a person whose pain is unbearable and whose suffering is beyond human endurance.

There are no easy solutions to any of these problems, and this book does not intend to provide simple answers to complex situations. At the same time we cannot stand back idly in the face of so much suffering. Our sense of responsibility and Christian love demand that we journey with those in pain, give support or consolation to those who suffer, and attempt to understand better our own personal pain and suffering.

Growing Through Pain and Suffering offers practical, helpful suggestions about how we can show compassion for and give support to the suffering. Standard expressions and pious platitudes are not effective. Suffering is *personal* and asks for *personal* understanding and response. To be ef-

fective—as pastoral ministers or as friends—we need to respond to the *personal* needs of those who suffer.

This book examines the link between suffering and the
individual's personality structure. This is done because
people react to suffering in the same way they react to life,
that is, according to what their own personality structure
allows.

Without becoming overly technical this book uses Erik
Erikson's eight stages of human development to provide a
general insight into the needs and tendencies of diverse
personality structures. Understanding what motivates a
person can help us to respond more personally and more
effectively to someone who is suffering.

The book is written for chaplains, pastors, caregivers,
and anyone who deals with people who suffer. Family
members who are the primary caregivers for people who are
seriously ill, aged, or infirm will find many helpful ideas in
these pages. In addition, this book will be helpful for those
who suffer. A deeper understanding of their own condition
may provide them with the support and encouragement
needed to allow the unavoidable companion of suffering to
become a friend on the journey of life.

Acknowledgments

I am very grateful to students at Duquesne University, Pittsburgh, and at Barry University in Miami Shores, Florida, for their many frank and honest observations that helped me to express my ideas with greater clarity. I am also grateful to Sr. Agnes Cunningham, SSCM; Rev. John O'Grady, STD, SSD; Rev. Henry J. Koren, CSSp; Sr. Geraldine Grandpre, CSJ; and Sr. Judith Shield, OP, whose careful reading and useful remarks contributed much to the form and style of this book. Last but not least I am grateful to Twenty-Third Publications, especially to Neil Kluepfel and Tom Artz for their encouragement and support.

Contents

GROWING THROUGH

Pain
&
Suffering

Suffering—
Part of Being Human

Wherever we look, we see pain and suffering. Not a single society, nor even a single human being can avoid it completely. Yet it is not something anyone wants. Heaven knows how hard we try to escape it and eliminate it. The more sophisticated a society becomes, the less tolerant people are of suffering. Enormous amounts of money and time are spent on research to understand and fight diseases, to curtail suffering, and eliminate accidents and other avoidable tragedies.

If we want to advertise how attractive a city or county is to live in, we describe healthy conditions, excellent health care facilities, low crime rates, high standards of living, and low incidences of terminal diseases. We never mention how well people deal with suffering caused by illness, poverty, or crime. Yet as a hospital chaplain, social worker, member of a parish staff, or a person concerned about the people in one's neighborhood or family, we all encounter incredible courage daily.

From the beginning of history humans have searched for ways to avoid or to heal suffering. We stay in shape through jogging, walking, and other exercises as a way of avoiding illness and forestalling old age. There is an almost infinite variety of diets and guidelines that tell us which foods are good for our health.

No matter how careful we are about our health, we have to admit that prevention and medication are not the ultimate guarantees for protection against suffering. There is something else, something beyond our control. People refer to it as fate, luck, or divine providence. Even in a technological age we cannot totally control our lives and avoid all suffering and pain. This attitude is not much different from the mentality of an old African woman I baptized in a hospital some forty years ago. When I was about to leave she handed me an amulet. "Take this, Father. I do not need it any more. I want you to have it. As long as you have it, no lion will ever attack you."

I never had the courage (or faith) to test the amulet's effectiveness. It struck me, however, that whether we are rich or poor, sophisticated or simple, technologically advanced or living in a stone-age society, we all look for powers beyond human control to avoid misery and suffering. Willingly or unwillingly, we all admit that higher powers have something to do with human suffering. Some people call these powers "God." Others refuse to give them a name at all.

The creation narratives in the Book of Genesis contribute to the conviction that God is somehow involved in human misery. The threat of evil loomed over humanity from its very beginning: "If you eat from this tree you will die" (Gn 2:17). The happiness of the first human being in the Garden was incomplete: "It is not good for the human person to be alone" (Gn 2:18). There was an innate need for a companion "of equal dignity." As soon as this companion of equal dignity was created and human existence seemed finally complete in the male-female relationship, another danger threatened human happiness. The devil, in the form of a serpent, deceived the couple. As a result suffering became a central and permanent part of human life (Gn 3:14–19). Humanity is thus confronted with the enigma that suffering is experienced as *contrary to human wholeness*, while at

2

the same time as something inseparably connected with it.

Many books have been written about suffering: how to avoid it, how to cure it, how to deal with it or accept it, or how to see it as something that God wants us to endure. Suffering is often presented as something we must learn to accept from God's hand and turn into an instrument of grace and salvation. This book will not discuss any of these convictions in depth, but one must wonder why the same accident, illness, or personal tragedy devastates one person while another goes through it with relative ease. Why is it that one woman whose spouse dies can readjust to life within a reasonable period of time, while another equally intelligent and stable woman continues to be paralyzed by the loss several years later? It is more perplexing when both possess a deep, personal faith in God, and share many other common characteristics.

Why is it that one person who completely loses the hearing in one ear can smile and honestly say: "I'll just have to be the best one-eared listener the world has ever known," while someone else, equally intelligent and professional, in the same circumstances is convinced that his or her life is ruined? Whether you are pastor, neighbor, chaplain, or family member, these questions will puzzle you (or even haunt you) every time you try to console or guide a hurting, grieving person.

These and similar questions continue to plague me as teacher, counselor, friend, or chaplain whenever I meet someone who is suffering physically or psychologically. It is not enough for me to understand that human life is composed of seemingly contradictory and mutually exclusive aspects such as growth and decline, longing for wholeness and the experience of brokenness, and living in a material world while being called to a spiritual destiny. I am concerned about responding to people where they are and reaching them at the point where they need help.

This book was written as a source of guidance and insight into just these problems. I do not claim to have the answers. However, many years as pastor and teacher, counselor, friend, and chaplain have given me the opportunity for much thinking and studying, for praying and working with people in need. I share the results of these reflections with those who deal with suffering in themselves or in others.

Most of the examples and anecdotes throughout this book are from personal experience; others are from the experience of friends and colleagues. In certain instances, a person may think that his or her situation is discussed, but I assure you that in all cases I have changed and adapted names and circumstances. Not a single anecdote reflects historical accuracy; the privacy of patients and the confidentiality of communications are carefully protected.

Chapter One

Understanding Suffering, Understanding God

Suffering does not exist in the abstract. There is always a particular individual or community who experiences suffering. Often there is a recognizable reason for it, such as an accident or food poisoning. Frequently there is a human cause, such as overactivity or drunkenness, injustice or violence. Sometimes there are other causes totally beyond human control, such as earthquakes or hurricanes. Sometimes an illness baffles individuals and medical experts. Whatever the reason or the cause, suffering will touch every one of us at some point in life. It will touch each of us in our own particular way, according to our own particular sensitivities, and according to the structure of our personality.

Suffering is a very personal experience. Quite often we do not know where it comes from, what it will mean, or where it will lead us. Frequently it changes our life-situation and demands a new and different response to our everyday living. It is often difficult to grasp its meaning. Many well-intentioned people try to give their own interpretation to the significance of a specific illness for a specific person, but this is frequently inaccurate and rarely gives any consolation.

Once when I was visiting a patient on my usual hospital rounds, I could not help overhearing a conversation between a clergyman and a patient (his parishioner) behind the dividing curtain in a multi-bed hospital room. The cleric reminded the patient in strong terms that this illness was not just a haphazard event, but a clear sign from God that it was time for this man to change his life. The pastor said that if the patient did not take this opportunity, he might not get another chance to make his peace with the Lord. The clergyman went on in this vein for a considerable time. In fact, there was not much of a conversation; I never heard the patient's voice.

After the visitor left, I looked, with some hesitation, around the curtain and found an elderly gentleman in utter distress. We started a conversation. He was brought in for a heart problem and had to take it very easy. He seemed a gentle man who spoke caringly about his family and friends. He was not a church-goer but he did believe in God and he did pray. At this moment he was very, very frightened.

It was not my task to judge the behavior of the pastor, but deep inside I was angry. "Why can we not take people where they are?" But then I thought, "Where are they?" and "Who determines that?" or "What are our criteria for evaluation?" It gave me much to think about.

The patient, let's call him Andrew, was not in any physical pain at that moment, but there was a severe psychological and perhaps spiritual pain. He was suffering intensely with the kind of suffering that occurs when a person not only is aware of his discomfort, but realizes its impact on his life. In this instance, he was agonizing about his relationship with God.

Andrew's condition demonstrates the difference between pain and suffering.[1] It is a clear illustration of the difference between the awareness of physical discomfort (i.e., pain) and the disturbing demands that the uncomfortable condition make on a person's life.

Andrew knew how precarious his condition was. He was warned that strong emotions could result in additional physical damage to his heart. No matter how much he tried to stay calm, however, the pastor's words caused great agitation. He was deeply confused because he had been quite satisfied with his life and considered himself a decent person —until the pastor pointed out how immoral he had been.

The heart attack and hospitalization were sources of considerable suffering for Andrew. He had always used his talents as well as he could in everyday life. He was grateful to God and told God so every day. The hospitalization and the inability to be physically active were sources of suffering. While suffering physically because of his heart condition, he also suffered psychologically because of his inability to care for his wife and children. Now a whole new dimension of suffering was added when he was told that his life was not acceptable to God.

The Many Dimensions of Suffering

Andrew's experience teaches us two things about suffering: first, that it can and does take place in various dimensions and on various levels of human existence, and second, that there is a connection between these various dimensions and levels.

Suffering is never merely physical. Every physical experience influences our ability to react to demands or expectations. Andrew's heart attack changed the way he expressed his loving concern for his family. He saw himself in a different light than he did before, and he had to adjust his self-image. This led to emotional and psychological turmoil, which had the potential of seriously impacting his physical health.

Understanding the intimate relationship between physical and psychological well-being is very important in the supportive care of the sick. Their physical pain influences their approach to life. For care to be effective, caregivers need to understand the personality structure of the patient. The personality is not just a quality in the individual. Experts in psychology point out that "the personality is the totality of inherited and acquired psychic qualities which are characteristic of one individual and which make this individual unique."[2] These psychic qualities constantly interact with physical qualities. They are influenced by physical condition and are partly shaped by them. Psychic and physical qualities form a unity that is unique for a specific individual. The following chapters will discuss this interaction in much greater detail.

The spiritual dimension of human life is another important factor in determining the way people understand and are affected by suffering. Most people accept the fact that there is a spiritual aspect in human life. They may call it "soul" or "spirit" or give it another name. This spiritual aspect expresses itself through the psychological qualities of intellect and emotions which make it difficult to recognize the spiritual aspect as a value in its own right. From this perspective religious topics are seen as the object of psychological functions, and via these functions influence human life. Just as the dream to become a great musician can totally preoccupy a person's thinking and acting, so also can the thought of the greatness of God influence and direct a person's life. In this framework religion is one of the many values that shape human self-expression.

The religious aspect of one's personality carries great weight in determining a person's outlook and value structure. Just as the psychological dimension gives a distinctive quality to the bodily existence that makes this existence human, so also does the spiritual dimension give a distinctive quality to the psychological existence that bestows a special dignity upon a person. It creates a special wholeness.

This religious dimension is the awareness and acceptance of the fact that a power beyond human control influences human life. Whether or not this power is called "God," it shapes and directs human life.

Understanding God in Different Ways

Gordon Allport speaks about a "religious sentiment" that expresses itself according to the culture and personality structure of the suffering person.[3] In the face of suffering we see totally different approaches to religious values. We have all met people who broke a leg or an arm. One person says that God is punishing him, the second wonders why God ever allowed this to happen, and the third one sees it as a new challenge in her life to which she is asked (by God) to respond. The unique responses to the identical physical injury show three very different understandings of God's role in the accident, three very different ways of dealing with it, and three very different understandings of God and God's expectations. There is a need for a very different style of pastoral support in each case.

We are mistaken when we think that everyone understands God in the same way we do. In an earlier work I divided the human understanding of God into three major categories.[4] First I discussed *the magical understanding of God*. People with this understanding accept God's existence and see God's presence everywhere in the material world. For special reasons, at special places, or in special objects they see a protective or punitive presence of God. The African woman who gave me the amulet as protection from lion attacks has this magical understanding of God.

There are other examples of people who have a magical understanding of God. The African people with whom I ministered for many years faithfully sacrificed leaves to the spirit of the forest. Without such sacrifices they feared that they would never reach their destination without some unfortunate incident. Since I "forgot" such sacrifices, they performed them for me. Crossing a little mountain stream, they warned me not to put my travel-stick in the water while stepping from stone to stone for fear of hurting or offending the spirit of the river. They strongly believed in a spiritual/divine presence in the amulet, the tree, and the river. It was a very localized presence and largely restricted to these places or objects, but it was a very real presence of a very real god.

Westerners might think they have outgrown such superstitions until they realize their aversion to the thirteenth floor of a building and their hesitation about continuing their journey when a black cat has crossed the street in front of them. Even the Catholic use of medals and similar religious objects is not always free from the conviction of a "localized protective presence" of God.

Secondly, there is *the religious understanding of God*. In this perspective we accept that God is the ruler of everything and nothing happens unless God wants it to happen. If I stay healthy it is God's gift, if I get sick God wants it to happen (for whatever reason). This God demands the careful observance of rules and regulations. Transgressions are punishable and since God is also infinitely just, not a single transgression or good act will be forgotten.

This understanding takes God out of the localized material presence that we have seen in the magical understanding, but it places God high on a pedestal. This God is rather unapproachable and looks down on creation from the high heavens. This God is moved by petitions and good deeds, and angered by sins or transgressions. God's presence is experienced through actions of remuneration or punishment. From this perspective God seems more interested in adoration, obedience, and fear than in being a God who is loved unconditionally.

Finally there is *the dynamic understanding of God* in which God exists and is the source of all life. All life flows from God and is a form of *God's self-communication.* Every existing object, animal, or person participates in the divine being in its own way. The human person, created in the image of God, participates in God's self-expression in a special way. The human individual in his or her activities is not called to act *for the sake of God,* nor does God *act through the human person,* as if the person were an instrument in the hand of God. Rather, humankind is called to form *one principle of operation* with the creating and redeeming God. A human person is not so much to live "for God" as to live "with God" in every human self-realization.

This dynamic understanding of God sees God in every created being. God is not a localized presence that protects or punishes according to the presence or absence of actual reverence, nor is God the punishing or rewarding judge who hovers over every individual. God is the dynamic, life-giving source of all created existence. Through this dynamic presence God calls the human person to accept responsibility for one's own growth and development. This understanding acknowledges God's presence and influence in all that happens, but not as a measuring, calculating, rewarding, or punitive God. It is the God who is always "self-expressing" but allows humanity to be the form in which divine love and concern are made visible.

Years ago a professor told me that the word "Yahweh" does not really mean "I am who am" but rather "I am the one who is continually expressing myself." It struck me how this translation attributes a dynamic nature and presence to God. By granting intelligence and free will to human beings, God offers them a special share in the divine life. God calls humanity to be the visible and tangible translation of the divine love in created existence.

These three general approaches to the understanding of

God hardly exist anywhere in their pure form. Almost always there is something of each approach in an individual's understanding of God, but quite often one of the forms is predominant. When such a predominant form manifests itself in a patient, a chaplain may not ignore it; nor may a caregiver respond from a totally different understanding of God. That would be like using the same words while speaking a totally different language.

The understanding of God is personal for every individual and is closely related to cultural and personal backgrounds. The more one understands the suffering person's personality characteristics and understanding of God, the better one will be able to respond to his or her needs in times of physical or emotional pain. This does not mean that every generous individual who visits the sick is supposed to be a professional counselor. A basic understanding of the human personality structure, and of what a person *might* feel in such circumstances, however, does provide a better possibility for understanding the person and journeying more effectively with the patient through the painful process of coping with illness or searching for wholeness.

Notes

1. James G. Emerson, *Suffering: Its Meaning and Ministry* (Nashville: Abingdon, 1986), p. 21.

2. See Robert Goldenson, *Encyclopedia of Human Behavior* (New York: Doubleday, 1970), II, 945 ff.

3. Gordon Allport, *The Individual and His Religion* (New York: Macmillan, 1949), p. 2 ff.

4. Cornelius van der Poel, *The Search for Human Values* (Mahwah, NJ: Paulist, 1971), pp. 16-20.

Chapter Two

Suffering and Self-Awareness

Understanding the human personality is not an easy task. We see only what the individual displays in activities and in reactions to circumstances of life. Based upon this information we may draw conclusions, but we must be very careful and remember that we are often guessing. All persons have their own pattern of behavior that sets them apart from others. Some patterns are so strong that one can predict quite accurately how an individual will respond under certain circumstances. Oldham and Morris state:

> Your personality style is your organizing principle. It propels you on your life path. It represents the orderly arrangement of all your attributes, thoughts, feelings, attitudes, behavior and coping mechanisms. It is the distinctive pattern of your psychological functioning—the way you think, feel, and behave—that makes you *definitely* you.[1]

The individual nature of the human personality is partly innate since genes are transferred from parent to child at conception. Many individual characteristics, however, are developed in very early human experiences. I remember hearing about a six-week-old baby girl who was brought to the Catholic adoption agency of a major city. The little child was clean and seemed well cared for, but as soon as a human hand touched the infant, she froze. Studying the child's background they found out that as a newborn, the infant was literally placed as a foundling at the doorstep of a social agency. The baby lived in six different foster homes in the six short weeks of her existence. She had experienced care, but not love, and now the little one froze whenever a human hand touched her.

It took a loving adoptive couple with the help of a psychiatrist about nine months before the little girl began to react to them in normal ways. Somehow the child had experienced that the care she received was not the result of being loved for her own sake. Being reduced to an object of care, however well intended, instead of being loved for her own sake, created mistrust rather than trust in the human surrounding.[2]

The early developmental stages put a mark on the behavioral pattern of an individual. A child that is wanted and deeply loved has a much better chance to be self-respecting and self-accepting than an unwanted child. Such a person will also be better able to reach out to others in loving ways.

Stage One: Basic Trust vs. Basic Mistrust

Children know whether they are loved for their own sake or for someone else's benefit. The experience of Matthew shows this clearly. Matthew was the third child of immigrant parents. When the parents arrived in this country the oldest child attended grade one, the second started kindergarten, and Matthew was a baby of two months. Both parents were well educated. The husband spoke English, but the wife knew only her native language. They were a hard-working couple with a deep love for their children. During the day the husband was at his office, the two older children were at school, and the wife was home alone with Matthew. The youngster assumed a very important place in his mother's life during the long and lonely "working hours."

When Matthew was about three years old he developed bed-rocking. While sound asleep in his crib, he rocked himself with such force that the crib literally moved through the room. The pediatrician did not seem to find it too serious a problem and assured the parents that he would outgrow it. When the time came for kindergarten, Matthew found it difficult to be away from home so long, but he managed. First grade was a different story. He refused to go with the other children, and when put on the school bus, he escaped and returned home in the shortest possible time. His mother took him back to school in her car and handed him (kicking and screaming) to the principal and the first grade teacher. With the permission of the parents the principal called in the school psychologist.

The psychologist asked Matthew: "If you could be any animal, what animal would you choose to be?" Without hesitation he answered, "A porcupine." The psychologist then asked, "Why a porcupine?" Matthew responded, "Then I can put up my pins and nobody can touch me." The psychologist told this story to the parents, and one day they asked me, "Why would Matthew say this? We have never treated him badly or unfairly in any way. We love him dearly."

I was a rather close friend of the family and had seen their love and care on many occasions. I assured them that I was convinced of their love, but asked the mother what language she spoke when she came to this country and with whom she could converse. She responded, "Only my native language. I could not really speak with anyone except with my husband and children." I then asked, "What did you do when your husband was at his office and the older two children were in school?" "I was alone with Matthew," she replied. "Thank God for Matthew. Without him I would have gone crazy."

I told her to recall those early days in this country and asked, "Between you and Matthew, who needed whom the most?" She pondered my question for a moment and then said, "I don't know. I think that I needed him as much as he needed me." "I think you are right," I said, "but tell me very honestly, do you think it is fair that a two-month-old child must support an adult person? Are you surprised that he now wants to put up his pins so that no one can touch him?" "My God, what have I done?" she exclaimed.

I assured her that she had done what any intelligent and loving mother would have done under those circumstances. There was no need to apologize or to blame herself. All that was important now was to address this situation and move forward. Supported by the parents' new insights and loving guidance, Matthew grew up to be an effective university professor, a dedicated husband, and a loving father who does not have the slightest need to put up his pins so that no one can touch him.

This story offers many valuable insights. It provides a clear example of the first of Erik Erikson's eight stages of human development: Basic Trust vs. Basic Mistrust. Basic trust is the experience of unconditional acceptance. Basic mistrust is exhibited in the continuous need to fend for oneself and to prove one's value, because no one offers an unconditional loving welcome. Such a person will find value in achieving or pleasing in order to be accepted.

Matthew experienced love from the earliest stages of his life, but this love was not unconditional. He had to be the emotional support for his mother. His personal value was intertwined with usefulness. Matthew found his personal value only in taking care of his mother. No one else was allowed to do anything for her. This was his exclusive terrain. He could never go to school for a whole day and leave his mother alone.

As Matthew's parents began to understand the dynamics of this situation, they provided occasions for Matthew to develop a healthier self-image based upon an internal and personal value. He learned to give and to care freely without thinking that he had to do this in order to earn acceptance. If the attitude of earning acceptance had not been intercepted at this early stage, Matthew could have grown up to be a very possessive individual for whom love meant to possess and to control. The story also demonstrates that an early developmental process can be re-directed and that early mistakes can be healed.

Learning Basic Trust and Self-Acceptance

A lack of self-acceptance and the desire to earn acceptance through activity and success is not always evident in the early stages of life. Sometimes it takes an accident to reveal it. This was the case with James who was a highly trained, very effective heavy equipment engineer in road construction. He was a good provider who loved his wife and daughter. In an accident he lost his right arm. Physical healing was as complete as could be expected. Through rehabilitation and retraining he learned to work very effectively with one hand. In his own mind, however, he was a mutilated, handicapped individual, unfit for the job for which he was trained. His self-confidence and self-respect were gone. He was bitter and angry, and became unbearable toward his wife and daughter. He refused to see a counselor and kept wallowing in his own misery.

A friend asked me to visit the family and see if there was anything I could do for the wife and daughter. James was not very friendly during my initial visit, but slowly the ice began to break. He let his anger flow and revealed an unbelievably deep inner fear and pain of becoming useless. He worried that his life would be worthless if he could not do his job and provide for his wife and daughter. It took a lot of patience on the part of the counselor and a lot of courage on James' part, but finally he turned his eyes away from the arm that was not there in order to focus on his healthy arm. He began to realize that he had a value independent of his physical abilities. He did not have to wallow in the thought that he was a handicapped and mutilated engineer. He began to see himself as the most effective and best trained one-armed engineer the city had ever seen. He learned to recognize and acknowledge a personal value independent of his physical disability. He learned to see that even with one arm he was a whole person. He accepted himself as he was and worked with his capacities as they were at that moment of life and development. Only when he had reached this point did love and peace return to the family.

James resembles many of us who grew up in a competitive environment. No one will tell a child that success is the key to acceptance, but this idea develops very rapidly in the child's feelings. The awards that are presented and the applause that is given to those who succeed are clear proof of the importance of success as the means to be accepted and respected. James saw his success and value in physical strength and mechanical knowledge. No one could handle those big machines better than he. No one could repair them as well as he. In the accident he had not only lost his professional ability but also the source of his personal value and independence. All he could see was self-doubt and shame.

Stage Two: Autonomy vs. Doubt and Shame

This situation calls to mind Erik Erikson's second stage: Autonomy vs. Doubt and Shame. James' self-doubt was so deeply rooted that even the sincere and loving care of his wife and daughter could not overcome it. He experienced their love as demeaning and saw their care as a belittling of his poor, handicapped, powerless state. James' pain went far beyond a lost arm and impaired capacity. It rocked the deepest layers of his personality. Even the belief in God's understanding, forgiveness (if that were needed), love, and acceptance was ineffective. In his own mind James remained an unacceptable loser. Only the (re-)discovery of personal value and dignity, independent from any success, enabled James to face himself, his family, and God.

In situations like this the concerned minister does not have to be a professional counselor. It suffices to be a sensitive person who can recognize the human source of pain.

Developing Sexual Self-Awareness

Growing up has many pitfalls. Not the least of them is the developing awareness of being a male or female. From a very early age children will imitate or play-act what they see adults do. They see the love of their parents and relatives, and they discover that people who love each other deeply are usually married. Children want to play-act this. Whenever they get punished for it, this punishment will touch the deepest layers of their self-respect and self-acceptance as boy or girl, as man or woman.

I experienced an interesting example of this when a four-year-old niece said to me, "Uncle, I want to marry you." I responded by saying, "Well, Suzie, that is very kind of you, but don't you think that you are too little to get married?" "Oh, but I'll grow up," she assured me. "I am sure you will, but can you do all the work in the house?" As she pondered this question I suggested, "How about waiting until you are much bigger? Then we'll talk again about it." She agreed and went off to play somewhere else.

I forgot all about the conversation until an hour or so later when someone tapped my shoulder. It was my niece, standing behind me on a chair. "Uncle, am I big enough now?" she asked. I joked with her by saying, "You are cheating, Suzie; you are not that big yet." She laughed, jumped off her chair, and ran outside happy and playing.

It would have been so easy to stop the conversation right at the start and to chide her for the inappropriate question, but that might have harmed her. Somewhere she had picked up the idea that when a girl loves a man they get married. For her there was nothing inappropriate about the question. She just wanted to tell me that, at the moment, I was her favorite uncle and that she loved me. Had I chided her, she could have felt rejected as a girl. She would have felt this deep within herself. If this kind of rejection happens too often, children (as well as teens and adults) may lose their self-respect and their sense of self-value as a man or a woman.

One of the more tragic examples I encountered was 17-year-old Kathy who was rushed to the hospital because of an overdose. Sitting at her bedside I remarked: "Life must have been very difficult for you before you decided to take the overdose." That simple statement opened the flood gates. She let it pour out how nobody cared for her and never had cared for her. From the time that she was a little girl people had teased her that she was ugly, and that nobody would ever marry her. Now for a second time a boyfriend had broken off a relationship. She felt that she could not go through life like this.

It would have been little consolation for Kathy if someone were to tell her that there are many more boys around and that at some point the right prince-charming will turn up. She was not interested in hearing that there were many more boys available. Nor did she care to know that suicide was an offense against God, and that God was always there to help her. All that Kathy experienced at that moment was the deep pain of personal rejection that made life unbearable. In the midst of her developing womanhood, she was rejected as a woman.

As ministers we must respond to people's pain, understand the destruction of their self-value, support them as precious individuals, and guide them slowly to a self-acceptance that is based on inner values.

Stage Three: Initiative vs. Guilt

Both Suzie and Kathy show the importance of the third Eriksonian stage: Initiative vs. Guilt. In this stage of human development individuals either experience a personal and inner value or the lack of these qualities. If Suzie had experienced rejection she would have felt guilty for doing what she thought was the nicest thing she could do. It would have contributed to a *sense of essential guilt:* She would have felt guilty for being the person she was. That is what happened to Kathy. She felt so guilty for being who she was that she felt life was not worth living anymore.

A chaplain, minister, or caregiver does not have to be a psychologist to help people face suffering like this. It is sufficient to be a sensitive person who can distinguish between a superficial disappointment and a deeply rooted flaw in the human developmental process.

Such flaws cannot be laid solely at the doorstep of the parents. The parents of Matthew and James were very intelligent and loving people. It was, rather, the circumstances of life and societal influences that played a significant role in the growth of their personalities. When the genuine love of his wife and daughter could not enable James to overcome his feeling of worthlessness, we can safely assume that there was a much deeper cause for his suffering than the loss of physical abilities. If healing does not occur at that deeper level, all the rest is only a band-aid. Kathy's pain could not be alleviated by pious sayings or prayers uttered by a hospital chaplain. She needed to experience a sense of personal value and self-worth before true healing could occur.

This chapter has focused on the first three stages of development as Erikson describes them. Further chapters will focus on other stages. Later on I will show how spiritual responses are closely related to the developmental stage from which the pain originated, and how, through proper response, we can guide patients to a human and spiritual wholeness.

Notes

1. John M. Oldham and Lois B. Morris, *Personality Self-Portrait: Why You Think, Work, Love, and Act the Way You Do* (New York: Bantam Books, 1990), p. 15.

2. In this chapter and the following chapters I will frequently refer to Erik Erikson's eight stages of human development. For more detailed study see Erik Erikson, "Identity and the Life Cycle," *Psychological Issues* (New York: International University Press, 1959), vol. I, n. 1.

Chapter Three

A Personal Response to Suffering

Our personality comes through in everything we do. We tend to act according to the way we are. Our personality is also evident when we face suffering. We tend to suffer according to the way we are.

James, the engineer mentioned in the previous chapter, acted as a well-trained, self-confident heavy equipment operator who found pride, personal value, and identity in his professional ability. When this ability was broken through an accident, his self-confidence, pride, personal value, and identity were broken as well. What was left was a person with a deep longing for professional autonomy and a nagging feeling of shame that he could not be what he wanted to be. He felt that he was no longer himself. His response was bitterness and anger. James acted and suffered according to a behavior pattern that he had learned as a child.

I am not implying that James was childish in his bitterness and anger. On the contrary, James was an intelligent and responsible adult who acted according to a behavioral pattern that had helped him since childhood. He had learned to experience acceptance, confidence, and value as a person (and as a professional) through the successful performance of duties and tasks. As long as he was able-bodied and healthy he experienced all the acceptance and confidence he needed. The attitudes and behavioral patterns that effectively protected him as a child and as a healthy adult, however, were no longer effective after his accident. It was in this time of crisis that their insufficiency became evident. Let's go back and reflect again on Erik Erikson's early stages of development.

Stage One Revisited: A Question of Acceptance

The first stage (Basic Trust vs. Basic Mistrust) tells us about the balance that is experienced when children are accepted unconditionally for their own sake, for the benefit of others, or when they are seen as a burden. Without any personal conscious awareness of it, children develop an undercurrent of self-acceptance and value, or the lack of it, according to the form of acceptance they experience. Any and all relationships will be filtered through this early experience. If the experience has been negative, a defense mechanism for self-protection and self-preservation will automatically spring into action. The foundling baby froze at any human touch because she knew herself only as an object to be cared for, not as a person to be loved. Little Matthew experienced himself as the source of support for his mother. He could not go to school and leave her alone all day. At the same time he resented the fact that he felt accepted for his mother's sake rather than for his own value, and so he wanted to put up his pins so that no one could touch him.

This basic sense of trust or mistrust forms a fundamental attitude that guides a person to act in a way that provides the person with the best balance in life and the most comfort and security. In an earlier study I have called this attitude a "criterion for mental health," because self-esteem and relationships with others, which form the basis of inner peace, will develop according to this basic tendency.[1]

Immediately connected with this criterion for mental health is another basic attitude which I call "the ethical modality."[2] This does not refer to the ethical value of an individual's activity. It rather describes the basic tendency according to which a person acts. It may also be seen as a personal frame of reference by which an individual will evaluate to what degree an action is acceptable. Thus Matthew had decided in his own mind that he could not stay in school all day and leave his mother home alone. It would have been a violation of the person he was—Mom's protector. Neither spanking nor severe words cured this. His attitude changed only when he came to know that he was accepted even when he could not be with his mother.

Obviously young children are not conscious of these tendencies. While these are instinctual reactions developed out of a sense of self-preservation or self-realization, they have, nonetheless, a deep influence on one's personality. Further development will strongly reenforce these tendencies unless a conscious effort is made to alter the way a child interacts with the people and events that touch his or her life for better or for worse.

Stage Two Revisited: A Question of Autonomy

There is no sharp dividing line between the first and the second psychosocial crisis of the Eriksonian table. The second crisis (Autonomy vs. Shame or Doubt) builds smoothly upon the first (Basic Trust vs. Basic Mistrust). The child that experiences love and unconditional acceptance at birth, will experience few problems when motor skills develop, and he or she advances from crawling to standing, from walking to running, and from admiring to touching the glittery vase on the table. A loving hand will always be nearby to guide the child.

Autonomy is an attitude that arises when children are

allowed to exercise their motor skills whenever and in whatever way they want. It is the security of being able to self-propel and act or investigate on their own. Sometimes this permission is not given and children get punished when they go where they are not supposed to go, or when they investigate and touch what they are not supposed to touch.

The irresistible urge to investigate and to experiment cannot be stopped. The natural urge to discover becomes a repeated (but unavoidable) source of punishment and a cause of humiliation for the child that is not accepted for his or her own sake. This irresistible urge becomes the source of shame and doubt about his or her own value. The results of this are visible in the child's attitudes toward daily life and behavior. Instead of a feeling of accomplishment the child will experience a feeling of shame and doubt about one's acceptability. Matthew's need to be his mother's protector became reenforced during his early childhood through the games he played with his parents. The play-help he gave was for him much more than play. It reflected one of his deepest needs and expressed the source from which his personal value arose.

In less favorable circumstances a child can become very rebellious and destructive. I remember a Christmas party at which one of the guests could not find a babysitter and brought her three-year-old son along with her. Not a minute would pass without her telling him, "Johnny, don't do this; don't touch that; don't go into that room." The more she corrected Johnny, the more impossible his behavior became. When it was time to open the Christmas presents Johnny violently tore the wrappings from his present. I could not help wondering *whom* he was tearing to pieces rather than *what* he was tearing apart.

The basic tendency that characterizes this stage of development is the opportunity or the lack of it to actualize oneself in the developmental process. The surrounding world is seen through the framework of the ability to cooperate willingly or to submit only to force. It is not difficult to recognize what was going on with Johnny. His parents' marriage had broken up shortly after Johnny was born. The young, immature mother gave little security to the newborn child and could not guide him in his earliest explorations. His developing personality was not allowed to activate itself. He was shamed and made to feel guilty with almost every step he took. At age three only threats and punishment could keep Johnny more or less in control. We can only guess how he will react as a young adult. I suspect that he will be a very difficult patient to work with, but what is worse, he will find it very difficult to be ill.

The whole mentality of such a person is geared to being on the offensive. Self-actualization could only occur to the extent that Johnny could fight his way through a particular situation. If circumstances did not go his way, he would lose self-control as well as self-respect. His whole framework of perception was focused on self-defense. He would cooperate only when forced to submit.

In everyday life negative qualities may not always be evident. They will become clear when such persons are ill or otherwise in need. The overflow of anger and the unwillingness to collaborate cannot be reasoned away or prayed away. It is necessary to understand the personality and its distortion from an early age before one can begin to re-build by offering support that touches the wounded core of such a personality.

Stage Three Revisited: A Question of Personal Worth

In the next stage of development Erikson speaks about Initiative vs. Guilt. The game play of my four-year-old niece, mentioned in the previous chapter, is only one example. If children are allowed to express their fantasies freely without the danger of rejection or ridicule, they develop a healthy sense of personal value and acceptance. They need not expect that their fantasies will always be fulfilled. The important point is that they are taken seriously as the persons they are. This sense of dignity, however unconscious it may be, allows them to be proud of themselves.

This sense of personal pride was painfully lacking in George, a gentleman of about fifty years of age. He had an insatiable hunger to be accepted. The slightest sign of approval caused him to cling to a person as if that person were his greatest benefactor. George would give the shirt off his back to please that individual. This need for approval made him very vulnerable. In an effort to please people, he made administrative and managerial decisions that got him into deep trouble with the law. George could intellectually see his mistakes. He made the best possible resolutions only to fall back into his old habit of pleasing people even at the cost of his own reputation.

George's background explains a lot of his needs. His mother resented being forced into marriage because she was pregnant. George was clearly an unwanted child. He was born prematurely and spent the first two months of his life in the hospital. Little bonding took place between mother and child during those crucial first weeks of his life. After he came home from the hospital he was cared for properly but did not experience love. His early steps toward independence were not guided in a loving way. He was uncoordinated and appeared awkward. George was not an aggressive child. He waited and longed for acceptance and love, but was afraid to reach out for it. Encouragement was rarely given. His father affirmed him occasionally, but only when they were beyond the reach of the mother's hearing. Praise was something that he always craved, but hardly ever experienced. He always felt guilty for what he did. He felt guilty for existing. No wonder that George irresistibly longed for acceptance and made serious mistakes seeking it.

In Erikson's third stage (Initiative vs. Guilt) we see the healthy development of a sense of personal inner-based value set against the lack of value and the need to experience value from external sources. I call this attitude a "criterion for mental health." All future activity and all relationships are colored by this undercurrent. The basic acceptability of all one's actions will be determined by the balance between the freedom of self-expression and the need to please others. George could easily understand how inappropriately he had acted when, in his need for friendship, he allowed himself to be manipulated into lending money to a smooth talker. He did not have the strength to avoid this trap in the future, however, until he dealt with this underlying tendency. This insight into the core of George's personality and the way it affected his actions was a first step toward healing, and a clear example of how people react to life according to their basic personality.

Stage Four: Industry vs. Inferiority

The first three stages focus on the individual primarily in the process of internal development. This development has its impact upon the person's external behavior but this impact is not always clearly evident at an early age. This impact begins to show a little more in the fourth stage of psychosocial development: Industry vs. Inferiority.

At the fourth stage a child gets in touch with reality. The fantasy period is over and the individual must test his or her wings in real life. The earlier learning took place mostly by osmosis, absorbing the perceived demands or expectations of one's surroundings so that life became as livable as it could be under the circumstances. When a child begins to attend school, he or she becomes more outward-directed and is expected to enter into the outside world by acquiring knowledge and by producing the results of the knowledge that is gained. Obviously, the influence of the past will remain very important. A basic self-respect and sense of personal value make it much easier to relate to the outside world than when a person feels unacceptable. The stage of industry vs. inferiority has precisely this form of acceptance—the acceptance of the product.

When children begin to attend school, the acceptance of the result of their work is closely related to their personal acceptance. Children that are ridiculed or rejected because of poor performance will begin to see themselves as inferior to others. To excel at least in one aspect can be a saving factor. James, the heavy machinery operator mentioned in the previous chapter, was not academically gifted, but he excelled in practical abilities. He experienced dignity and value in being good at shop classes and mechanics, and became an excellent engineer.

The underlying attitude in this fourth stage is the balance between the ability to work with a set of inner standards and the continued uncertainty of whether or not what one does is worthwhile. James' inner standards told him that he was good with his hands, particularly in working with mechanical equipment. That ability became his self-image. Unfortunately for James, it became the strongest, if not the only, positive self-image that he had. Consequently, James collapsed when he could no longer be the mechanic he wanted to be.

Something similar occurred in George who also did not have a strong inner sense of worth, and who drew his sense of personal value from the approval of others. He climbed the social ladder effectively, but could not handle the fact that someone might accuse him of being inconsiderate. In both James and George the experiences of their early development became characteristic of their future activities.

These first four stages of development describe in broad lines the basis for growth of the personality. They picture the development of inner attitudes and the first steps toward the interaction of the individual with the world of people and things. It is not appropriate for chaplains, caregivers, family members, and friends to function as counselors or to try to rebuild the personality of the person who is suffering. A general knowledge of these basic undercurrents is very useful, however, for better understanding the pains and needs of people with whom we work and whom we try to support or guide to integrate into their lives the conditions in which they find themselves.

The remaining four developmental stages described by Erikson focus more on adult attitudes toward life and the concrete ways that people live their lives and face the situations of pain and suffering that arise. Succeeding chapters of this book will describe these stages and the effect they have on a person's ability to cope with suffering.

Notes

1. See Cornelius van der Poel, *The Integration of Human Values* (Denville, NJ: Dimension Books, 1977).
2. *Ibid*, p. 61 ff.

Chapter Four

Suffering Through
the Stages of Growth

In previous chapters we have discussed how the early stages of development that take place during childhood have an impact on the way people cope with illness and adversity when they are adults. The first four stages of Erikson's theory of psychosocial development, however, give us only a very incomplete picture of a person's growth and development. While these stages are fundamental and provide the basis for further unfolding, the continuing growth process that takes place in the teen and young adult years often modifies childhood attitudes.

Individual psychosocial development is not uniform and can go in many different directions. Each personality structure will have its own characteristics, and no two people are the same. In our ministry with family members, friends, parishioners, or patients it is important to understand every individual as deeply as possible. The better we grasp the inner workings of a person, the more effective our ministry will be. Because of this it is important that we reflect on the next four stages of the human psychosocial development as outlined by Erik Erikson.

Stage Five: Identity vs. Identity Diffusion
At this stage an individual leaves childhood and begins the

mysterious road to adulthood. This particular stage has some similarity with the very first stage (Basic Trust vs. Basic Mistrust). Both stages mark the beginning of an unknown and unpredictable series of happenings. Leaving childhood and entering adulthood is not as simple as merely entering a different room and closing the door behind you. On the contrary, all the good and the bad of childhood comes with a person and influences every step of the way.

Physical growth takes place rapidly during this stage and will frequently cause an embarrassing awkwardness. Youngsters may bump their head at places where they used to pass freely. Their clothes don't fit too well any more. Life seems to be out of proportion. The smoothness of movement and gesture seems to have been lost. The body matures, and although the young people already know that they are a boy or a girl, they are not prepared for the strangeness of the physical and psychological feelings that accompany this new spurt of growth.

Young people who are outgrowing childhood want to be independent from their parents, yet at the same time, they are yearning for guidance on the puzzling road to adulthood. They are not and do not want to be little children any longer. They want to be adults, but they have no clue what that really means. They are like strangers in a strange land where the only safe company is the company of their peers.

Clashes between parents and teenagers are legendary and countless, but also understandable. While parents have some insight into the dangers of this period and want to help their children avoid the pitfalls of adolescence, young people need to try their own wings and be independent. The nature and form of the clashes depend largely on the existing parent-child relationship. These clashes will often reenforce the negative elements of the past while writing the script for the future. The case of Bert is an example of this.

Bert was sixteen years old and the oldest of five children. He displayed a complete indifference and lack of concern for anyone in the family. He could be very nice and cooperative when it was to his advantage, but he was impossible, insensitive, mean, and rebellious when that suited his needs. Bert was in a constant power struggle with his father who often used his belt to make Bert do what he wanted him to do or to punish him for transgressions of any kind. Bert's mother seemed to keep a distance and one never knew which side she was on. Sometimes she sided with the father; at other times she seemed to protect Bert.

Bert's present attitude did not start when he was fifteen. It was in the making from his early childhood. His father was in the armed forces, and while he did not have a high military rank, he was the commander-in-chief at home. His wife put up with it reluctantly most of the time, but occasionally she expressed her resentment. They had very different ideas about education and formation. The father believed strongly in military style discipline; the mother was inclined to give in whenever the children needed something. The children got many mixed messages.

Bert entered his teenage years with a poor self-image and a serious doubt about whether he could do anything right. He tried hard to set himself free from his parents, but they did not allow him to be away from home for any length of time. The more they insisted on obedience, the more Bert fought for his freedom. Verbal abuse, corporal punishment, and fisticuffs with his father were common occurrences.

It is obvious that explanation and encouragement were not very effective in these circumstances. To deal with Bert's anger and inappropriate behavior it was necessary to recognize what had happened at the earliest stages of development. Bert felt that he could not trust anyone and that he had to fight for everything. His perception of reality was seriously distorted and he felt that he had to prove himself to himself and to others. There was little sense of personal value and dignity.

A sense of personal value and dignity is exactly what a young person needs and wants to find in adolescence. If a person does not find these qualities, he or she will enter into adulthood with a lack of purpose or with the deep insecurity of the teenage experiences. In this case the young person will be forced to face adult life with an immaturely developed emotional system.

Stage Six: Intimacy vs. Isolation

At this stage all the experiences of childhood and young adulthood blend together to form a personality that can face, independently and responsibly, all that life has to offer. The major positive characteristic of this stage is intimacy—the ability to love. People with a well-developed sense of intimacy can relate to others without fear of rejection. They possess the ability to relate constructively and in depth to others without the need to control or the urge to hurt.

People with a healthy sense of intimacy allow themselves to be known in depth by others without fear of rejection. To be known is to be vulnerable, and intimacy allows people to be vulnerable. Healthy intimacy enables people to face their own strengths and weaknesses without being afraid of them, and accept the strengths and weaknesses of others. They have the courage to allow their own strength to flow over into the other without fear of losing it. They can form with others a unit of cooperation for mutual growth and happiness. Whenever that self-acceptance is missing, however, people will either isolate themselves or use others for their own fulfillment and wholeness. Two examples of young couples in love will show the difference that intimacy makes in people's lives.

Judy and Louis were an interesting young couple. Judy was a lively, intelligent, healthy young woman. Louis handled, with some effort, a motorized wheelchair. Their reason for seeing me was clear and direct. "We would like to get married and the bishop sent us to you, since you are the Family Life Director for this diocese." I asked them to tell me why the bishop sent them to me, and learned that shortly after their engagement, Louis had broken his neck in a diving accident. He was paralyzed from the neck down. Judy, an executive secretary, spent all her spare time with him in the hospital after the accident. Louis, for his part, tried as hard as he could to get her out of his life. During visiting hours he was unpleasant and outright nasty to her, telling her bluntly to get out of his life. He told her that she was young, attractive, and competent. He felt that his body was broken, his life was ruined, and he had nothing to offer her. He wanted them to break off the engagement so that she could date other people and build a future. Judy's response was that she never loved him just because he had a healthy, athletic body, but because of the person he was. She felt that this person remained, even after the accident.

Encouraged by her unwavering confidence and concern, Louis worked hard at his physical therapy. He learned to handle a motorized wheelchair and even learned to drive a van with adapted steering. He enrolled at a community college and studied accounting. Everything was going very well for Judy and Louis until they went to the pastor of their parish to register for marriage. The pastor had serious reservations against the marriage of a healthy young woman and a paraplegic. He told them that their case was special and that they should see the bishop. The bishop listened to them with much compassion and interest, and then told them to see the Family Life Director.

We had a long conversation that first evening. They came back for a second and a third time. Throughout these conversations I gained a good insight into their personalities. The more I learned about them, the more I admired and respected them. Rarely had I seen such a degree of maturity in young people. Louis was very much aware of his limitations. He had no unrealistic dreams about his future. Both of them had devoured all the literature they could get on paraplegia. Louis could offer Judy love and dedication in his limited way. Judy, for her part, was not acting out of a false sense of guilt because the accident happened in her family's swimming pool, nor was she driven by an unhealthy feeling of compassion or pity. She knew the limitations that Louis' paraplegia would put on her, but she recognized his value as a person and offered him respect and love. Both were convinced that they could be a source of personal growth for each other.

After further necessary inquiries I suggested that they tell their pastor that I did not see any objection to their marriage and that I would call him personally to discuss the marriage. Leaving my office they stopped at the door and said, "Father, it would mean so much for us if you would perform our wedding." The wedding was special and different. The most impressive moment for me was when Louis had to sign some papers. In a very clumsy way he put a brace over the fingers of his right hand, found a little stump of a pencil which he positioned in his hand, and signed his name with the same clumsy effort that a little boy in kindergarten would use to sign his name. During this whole process Judy was watching him with all the patience in the world. She was perfectly content to let him do this on his own. They were able to love, and they were open to sharing each in their own way. Tragedy had taught them a lifetime of wisdom in a very short time. This event happened many years ago. They still keep in touch. They seem to be happy and have an adopted family.

How very different was the case of Martin and Sheila. Their pastor sent them to me to evaluate their readiness for marriage. At my invitation they sat down and I asked them to tell me something about themselves. Sheila slouched back in an easy chair while Martin sat up and led the conversation. He did not talk about himself but explained in great detail how strict and unreasonable Sheila's parents were. He explained that Sheila was not allowed to do anything on her own, and that she really needed to get away from home to a place where she could develop her talents. At some point I interrupted and said, "Sheila, what do you think about all this?" Sheila came up from her slouched position and just when she opened her mouth to speak, Martin made one little gesture that made her recline back into her chair while Martin continued to explain how he would make her free. I was not overly convinced.

Further conversation showed that I was dealing with two immature individuals. Martin had the irresistible need to control somebody else's life in order to feel a sense of power and importance. Sheila could not exist without an authority that controlled her. She was more than tired of her parents' control, so Martin would be much better. At first sight they fit together like a hand in a glove. Nonetheless I advised them to postpone their marriage for a while and get some help. Two immature individuals do not make a mature couple; they form a marital disaster in the making.

Martin and Sheila had never faced themselves. They only experienced their needs, and from their needs they reached out to each other. Each one could fill the emptiness in the other, but they could not enrich each other or heal each other's immaturity. They would cling to each other as long as it suited them, but the poverty of their relationship would soon manifest itself. They would probably end up in bitter fights and deep unhappiness. They could not give from the richness of their being, but they would grab whatever they could and appropriate it to themselves to fill their own incompleteness. They were inclined to hang onto what they had and carefully guard their own interests.

These two examples help us to understand the meaning of intimacy and isolation. They show the difference between generous reaching out and anxious self-protection, and illustrate clearly the two major ways of reaching out in daily human relationships. One is an attitude of generously sharing one's own richness so that both persons can grow to greater depth. It leads to greater freedom and independence so that each partner can decide in freedom to love the other. We see this in Louis and Judy who wanted to share rather than to appropriate. The other attitude of reaching out results from the couple's own poverty. The need to control and the need to be dependent reflect a lack of true personal value. Martin and Sheila need each other to complement their own personality. Their relationship is not based on an intimate sharing, but on an unhealthy taking in order to possess. In living out these needs people usually grow poorer and needier as time goes on.

Stage Seven: Generativity vs. Stagnation

When Erikson spoke of generativity, he was not referring to procreation. Generativity is the human ability to give of oneself for the development, growth, and happiness of another. If the major characteristic of intimacy is the ability to love, the primary perspective of generativity is adequacy in interpersonal relationships. Such persons have a sense of personal security that allows them to be sufficiently assertive without being offensive or overly aggressive. They trust other people but strongly resist being manipulated. They can reach out to others for the sake of others and for their own enrichment, but will not cling to others or try to control them. When this openness and generosity are not present, a person will have poor interpersonal relationships and often try to control others.

The marriage of Bill and Anne was an interesting, but sad, example of stagnation and a lack of generativity. Bill had been married before but the marriage broke up because of his wife's infidelity. Now he had married Anne who was a quiet, hard-working, family-loving lady. Bill was very thoughtful and generous to her. Without any particular reason he might come home with flowers, take her out to dinner, or go shopping with her. He would buy her whatever she wanted. Money was no problem. The problem, however, was that he would not allow her to go anywhere by herself. She could not even go out alone to visit her mother, or go window shopping with a girl-friend. At irregular times during the day he would call her from work to say "hello," but really to check up on her. If he ever caught her absent all hell would break loose. He told her very bluntly: "You will never play the trick on me that my former wife played." It did not take very long before Anne did play the same trick on him. The marriage did not last many years. Counseling was ineffective since Bill was immovably stuck in his need to control and filled with deep-seated suspicion.

Somewhere in his growth process Bill had developed a deep mistrust in himself. He could not accept the fact that anyone could love him and be faithful to him. For him loving was equated with buying gifts. He could only offer this form of happiness, and he needed to stay in control of the relationship. Any social relationships that he could not control would not be tolerated. He had totally isolated himself socially and he demanded the same from his wife. He was so stuck in his past that he could not allow himself to develop as a person. Nor could he allow personality development in his wife. He could not accept partnership, only servitude. Bill's whole relationship was characterized by a fearful protecting of himself and all that belonged to him. The chances for further development and growth were minimal.

Stage Eight: Integrity vs. Despair or Disgust

The human growth process is like a mosaic composed of innumerable little pieces; very insignificant on their own, they all contribute to the beauty of the total picture. Every activity, every experience, every success, and every disappointment contributes to the formation of the individual. In favorable circumstances people learn to face up to all the demands of life, and learn to handle themselves well even in the most trying situations.

Not all people cope with life in the same way, however. Some can handle anything that comes their way. Then there are others who struggle with the smallest of life's trials and tribulations. Even when only a few pieces of their personal mosaic are out of place, the whole picture loses much of its beauty and value.

Many people find life especially difficult when they enter mid-life. After surviving childhood, teen, and young adult years, they feel like they should finally be able to stand on their own feet. Life should run smoothly and their goals should be clear. Instead they experience emptiness and insecurity. They do not know what direction to go. The dreams they had in their youth have not materialized and they have lost the interest and energy to seek after new dreams. There is a sense of despair as they search for a foothold from which they can tackle life. There is also a feeling of disgust because they have not succeeded in finding a clear direction for their own life despite many years of study and work.

Gerald's situation is typical of the mid-life struggle of many people who seek to maintain a sense of personal integrity and avoid serious doubt or despair. As a young priest Gerald was assigned to missionary territories and did his work quite well. He was loved by his parishioners and respected by his confreres. He did so well that, in his early forties, he was elected provincial superior in a very difficult missionary territory. He remained successful until, at a certain moment, he seemed to lose hold of his life. He became despondent, fearful, insecure, and self-effacing. His self-esteem was so low that he refused to seek help because he felt that he did not deserve it.

In counseling sessions Gerald told his counselor of an incident from his teen years that shed some light on his present behavior. Gerald wanted to become a priest but his father was not happy about his decision. After resisting for a long time, the father gave in. At the age of thirteen Gerald went to a high school seminary far away from home, where he almost died of homesickness. Within four weeks he ran away from the seminary and came back home. His father gave him a tongue lashing that devastated Gerald, but he never spoke about it again. He tried hard to forget it. Within a year, however, he wanted to go back to the seminary. After some negotiating he was allowed to attend a nearby high school seminary as a day student. From then on everything went smoothly, and he completed college, novitiate, and theological studies without any problems.

His career as a priest was successful and yet he never completely overcame the inner pain caused by his father's verbal castigation. He saw himself as his father had pictured him some thirty years earlier, but he had never really dealt with those feelings. He had suppressed them effectively through hard work and dedication, but deep down he still saw himself as the good-for-nothing, undecided, lazy individual, exactly as his father had portrayed him.

Gerald slowly restored his self-image, began to accept himself again, and saw clearly the positive results of his labors. The mosaic of his life had a flaw which had to be repaired before inner peace and happiness could be found. He regained his efficiency in handling everyday situations and found new direction in his life. He developed an integrity and wholeness in which the structure of his life took an acceptable shape. He acknowledged his strengths and his weaknesses and learned to respect himself in this process.

While these examples of the various stages of development are extremely brief, they give some insight into the complexity and beauty of the human personality. Although you may wonder what all this developmental theory has to do with pastoral care and support in illness, these theories are extremely relevant. Remember that human beings act and react according to their personality. They face suffering and pain based on the way they have become through circumstances of life and through personal involvement in their own growth processes.

When illness strikes and disables the normal functioning of the individual, it usually throws the person back on an earlier defense mechanism. A healthy early self-image will offer a solid basis for readjustment; a poor early self-image may make readjustment very difficult. Illness, tragedy, and suffering may cause the disintegration of the personality, but they may also offer a challenge for growth. Succeeding chapters will explore the personal and spiritual challenges faced by people who are suffering, and the potential for growth offered by illness, tragedy, and pain.

Chapter Five

Suffering—
From Disintegration to Growth

The developmental process of the human personality suggests an almost infinite number of possible human responses and an endless variety of attitudes toward pain and suffering. In seemingly identical circumstances two people may react entirely differently. The same verbal offense that drives one person into a violent rage, makes another person crawl into a shell, while still another shrugs it off as insignificant. The same physical illness sends one person into a deep depression, while another takes it in stride. Anyone who deals with patients suffering physical or emotional illnesses will encounter these different responses frequently, if not daily. One is often at a loss as to how to deal with such individuals or with their various mood swings.

It helps to remember that all responses are expressions of an individual personality under specific circumstances. The nature of the physical or emotional hardship is obviously an important factor in the human response. No less important, however, is the meaning of the hardship for the particular individual. Joseph Fichter, quoting Clifford Geertz, points out that the problem of suffering is an "experiential challenge in whose face the meaningfulness of a particular pattern of life threatens to dissolve into a chaos of thingless names and nameless things."[1]

In daily experience, suffering is not only a hardship. It quite frequently tears the personality to pieces. Normal activity becomes difficult or may be totally impeded. One's usual strength ebbs away. Efficiency is reduced to a minimum. While this behavior is understandable, it is not universal. Where illness or an accident cause a disintegration in certain persons, a similar experience may challenge others to an expression of almost superhuman strength and courage.

Strong Faith, Strong Personality

Joe and Mary were a happily married couple with four adult children. One evening as they were returning home from a visit to friends, a truck being driven by a drunk driver crossed the median strip and crashed head-on into their car. Mary was killed almost instantly. Joe was rushed to the hospital in very serious condition. The hospital staff and the children were faced with the difficult task of informing Joe of his wife's death. Initially they did not approach this topic, but Joe began to ask about Mary. In view of the seriousness of Joe's condition, the medical staff suggested hiding the truth for fear that Joe might lose his will to live.

Aware of Joe's alertness and sensitivity, the chaplain and the children took a different view. Step by step they informed Joe of the seriousness of Mary's injuries. They first assured him that she was well taken care of and that he did not need to worry about her. A day later the whole truth became clear to Joe. For a moment he seemed to collapse, but when his children said to him, "Dad, we need you now more than ever," he squeezed their hands and inaudibly mouthed the words, "We'll win." He joined his children in planning all the details of his wife's funeral. At the time of the funeral he was sad, but at peace. His recovery was unexpectedly fast, and he was able to return home for further recuperation until he was ready for more intensive physical therapy.

Faced with this kind of courage we cannot help wondering about the source of such strength. Joe was a deeply religious man, and his faith in God undoubtedly had a great influence on his attitude. But faith never works independent of the human personality.[2] Underneath his religious convictions was a personality structure that was capable of dealing with hardship.

Coming from a healthy family, Joe grew up with a sense of personal value. He did not have to prove himself through any pose of grandeur, through successful activities, or through pleasing people. He was able to reach out to others for their sake because he had something to offer from deep inside himself. Likewise he was able to receive praise without feeling embarrassed and without clinging to those who praised him. He could open himself up to others without fear or shame.

Joe's marriage to Mary was another source of affirmation. The two responded to each other in extraordinary ways, often sensing each other's presence or condition without words. This allowed them to become increasingly more independent as personalities who freely chose to be fully dedicated to one another.

Joe's grief over Mary's death was felt more deeply than any language can describe, but it did not break his personality. His physical health was precarious due to his own injuries. The loving relationship he had built with Mary was just a memory, yet he had the strength to continue the responsibilities that he and Mary had assumed together. Throughout his lifetime he had shared his own personality with Mary and the children, and in return he had accepted their love and self-giving for his own growth. The strength of their intimate friendship never left him. His present condition was a new challenge, not so much to prove himself as to reach out constructively to his children and to others. Perhaps because he was more sensitive than most people, he was also emotionally stronger than most people. His present suffering occasioned a new growth and a new depth of personality.

Finding the True Source of Pain

James and Sue were a very different couple. As explained in Chapter Two, James was proud that he could handle the heaviest of road building equipment with the same ease that a little boy can handle his toy trucks. This all changed when James lost his right arm in an accident. Physical care and retraining as a mechanic put him back on the job, but he was no longer the proud heavy equipment operator. He could handle some lighter machinery, and he did this with remarkable efficiency. In his own mind, however, he was nothing more than a handicapped, mutilated heavy equipment engineer who was downgraded to a lower class job. Anger and bitterness radiated from his whole being and made life for his family a living hell. Despite successful physical rehabilitation and retraining, James' life had effectively disintegrated.

To understand James' response to his accident, we need to analyze the underlying motivation that shaped James' response. He had always been a very reliable worker. He loved his wife and children. He was a faithful husband and a good provider, but his life changed radically after the accident. It is James' childhood that gives us some inkling of his inner needs and limitations. Although his family of origin was rather stable and loving, James had not experienced acceptance for his own sake. There was a continual need to prove that he was a person of value. Although his marks at school were only average, he excelled in practical knowledge and abilities, and he developed into an outstanding mechanic.

Without realizing it, James' self-esteem resulted more from professional success and physical prowess than from his inner value as a person. The love for his wife and children was sincere, but underneath this love lurked the fear that their respect for him was dependent on his success as a provider. He saw himself now as a prisoner of his handicap. This made him angry and bitter. Somewhere in the development of his personality was a distortion that prevented him from grasping his value as a person and integrating it into the fabric of his life and relations.

When his dream fell apart, he fell apart as a person. All he could see was the missing arm and the consequent inability to be the efficient engineer he once was and wanted to be again. Only when a counselor turned James' eyes away from the empty spot of the missing arm, and made him see his own personal value and his exceptional ability to be creative even with one arm, did he begin to change his perspective and develop into a highly effective one-armed engineer. Above all, he developed into a person with a deep self-respect who accepted himself as he was. Suffering had been a hard teacher and these lessons were painful for James, but he managed to journey through the pains of disintegration to a new discovery of personal wholeness.

I do not suggest that every supportive contact with people who suffer must take the form of a counseling or therapeutic relationship. Far from it. But if we are striving for a holistic healing process, one of the major requirements is to know where the pain comes from. The obvious source of pain is not always the deepest source.

As a result of the accident that killed his wife, Joe suffered from physical injuries that were painful and frustrating. A broken leg, broken ribs, and separated shoulder are serious obstacles to normal activity. The independent person becomes dependent, and the self-sufficient individual must rely on others. More serious was Mary's death. Joe's closest and most intimate friendship was cut off. An ideal and goal in life had been destroyed.

It is hard for the human mind to comprehend the magnitude of such pain, and yet, we cannot help Joe if we do not help him to deal with it honestly and openly. Joe experienced a very serious loss, and healing must respond to this loss. An important first question is, "What does physical independence mean for Joe?" From the early stages of his childhood Joe experienced a sense of personal acceptance and value. Although physical and professional success played an important role in his self-esteem, it was not its major source. It had more the character of an important affirmation. The loss of independence was painful, but an inner resilience enabled him to see his present condition as a new and different demand to exercise personal independence. His personality was not broken. Only the conditions under which he expressed himself had changed.

Similarly, we must ask what Mary's death meant to Joe. Did he lose a companion or a protector? Was he a man who found fulfillment in life primarily by caring for others; in this case, Mary and the children? If this were so, life would have lost its meaning. Or was Mary the person with whom he could share his inner depth and values, with whom he could grow and unfold his personal qualities? Did Mary contribute to his wholeness without replacing his inner self?

In each of these circumstances the wound of the loss is different, and effective healing has to correspond to the nature of the wound. Joe and Mary were close companions, but neither of them was an immature person who relied upon the other for completeness. Instead they reached out to each other for mutual growth and the unfolding of their personalities. This does not make the pain less intense, but it makes the consequences very different and asks for a particular healing approach and process.

James' accident showed another pattern. Unknown to himself, there was an identification between his professional abilities and his self-value as a person. The loss of his arm was more than the loss of the ability to work. The accident destroyed his self-esteem. Medical care had saved his life, but the self-image of the independent and proud engineer had died. Rehabilitation and professional retraining gave him the ability to work with one hand, but they did not restore his self-esteem. The care and support that were given were good and genuine, but they were limited to physical recuperation and retraining.

James' deepest wound, however, was not the loss of his arm and its consequent professional limitations. The deepest loss was the destruction of self-value or self-respect, and the consequent inability to relate confidently and lovingly to those who were close to him. The challenge that James faced went beyond professional retraining, and dealt with the rebuilding of his personality. Sue and the children were a major factor in this process. After his accident, he initially experienced their acts of love and dedication as expressions of sympathy and compassion toward an unfortunate, crippled man. Instead of comforting him, they reminded him of his limitations and added to his bitterness. Fortunately, James accepted the challenge to make personal changes. He learned to value his own inner self and took pride in what he was able to do with his one hand. His family's love became an important and constant affirmation, which he learned to appreciate and which contributed to his personal growth.

Understanding the Grief Process

The same principles of searching for the true source of pain and suffering must be applied when we are dealing with grieving families or individuals, or when we take care of persons with emotional problems. Let us first consider the problem of grief.

Grief can be a severe form of suffering.[3] It is not merely weeping about the loss of a person or object. Grief is the experience of a loss that affects the individual in the deepest layers of one's personality. It is a response to a loss which has its repercussions in the person's physical and emotional structure. Grief is the experience that something is torn away from one's being, and that one is left incomplete and disabled. The loss causes a new situation for the individual that sometimes demands a rebuilding of the personality.

Grief has two essential aspects: (a) a loss that affects the deepest layers of the personality, and (b) a process in which the individual restores his or her life to its original condition or readjusts to live effectively in the new situation. Both aspects are so closely interwoven that neither of them can be dealt with without dealing with the other. The circumstances surrounding Peter's death may serve as an example of this.

Peter and Elly were a happily married couple with a large family that lived together, played together, laughed together, and faced hardships together. They worked a family dairy farm in Europe, milked the cows, had their homemade dairy products, and lived a normal, thrifty life. Around the age of sixty Peter began to lose his strength, and began to have difficulty walking and doing strenuous work. His condition was later diagnosed as amyotrophic lateral sclerosis (Lou Gehrig's disease). Most of the care, including feeding and eventually suctioning when Peter could not cough up the mucus from his lungs, fell back on Elly. The family physician kept a close watch by making daily visits. Most of the time, however, Peter and Elly were on their own. One night the coughing became too much. Elly could not handle it. Before she could call for help, Peter died in her arms, suffocating on the mucus from his lungs.

Elly was inconsolable. She could not think, let alone speak about Peter's illness and death without bursting into tears. Yet she wanted to speak about it as if it were something that she had to expel from her system. Perhaps she needed to convince herself that she had no guilt in his death. Several years after Peter's death she still could not talk about it without breaking down in tears.

In analyzing this situation we see several significant points. First, Elly lost a husband who was a good provider, a supportive companion, and a caring father to their children. Much of the meaning of her life had fallen away. While most of the children were married and lived their own lives, the younger ones still needed a father's care and attention. Elly had to face this task alone. Although she came from a large family and had a large family of her own, she was indecisive by nature and had great difficulty making important decisions about her own life. She felt as if she were powerlessly swinging in the wind.

Second, Peter's long illness had brought them closer together. She had become the one who nurtured him, dressed him, fed him, and took him wherever he had to go. He filled her life and strengthened her mothering instinct. This condition fed strongly into Elly's strongest and weakest qualities. She was a nurturing person who was at her best when she cared for others. She had no difficulty letting her children go out on their own to build their own homes, but she lost her self-worth when she could not support the life that was entrusted to her. Peter's death wounded the core of her being. She had failed.

In addition, she was haunted by the thought that she had perhaps acted inappropriately and hastened his death. The vision of his agony was constantly in her mind. The indecisiveness of her personality played into her feelings of guilt. Intellectually she knew that she had done everything she could. There was no chance that Peter could have survived his illness, yet deep in her heart there remained the nagging uncertainty of, "What would have happened if...?" with many undefined possibilities.

Elly experienced Peter's death as more than the loss of a husband and the father of their family. The strength of her personality, the decisive direction of her life, and her nurturing ability were all shaken by his death. Her sense of honesty and responsibility was severely threatened by the fear that she had not called for help soon enough. Each of these factors influenced the nature of the process of grieving and of subsequent healing.

Elly's life can never return to its previous condition. She needs to adjust to the present situation. This readjustment requires first that she deal seriously with her own basic indecisiveness. She needs a stability and direction that come from her inner self. It is very difficult, however, to convince a mother of ten that deep down she needs to develop the ability for decision making, and that she has to develop greater personal independence and self-confidence. Yet this lies at the heart of her grieving process.

Once greater self-confidence is developed, it will become easier for her to deal with the guilt feelings that cause so much pain. A deeper sense of inner value, independent of external success, may enable her to see that even the best human efforts are not always sufficient to satisfy our desires. With self-acceptance at the core of her personality the readjustment to life can begin to take shape.

This process sounds very simple on paper. In the reality of human life, however, it is a long and painful struggle.

There is no way to force it or to accelerate it. Only sympathetic compassion and understanding combined with endless patience can help Elly to reconstruct her life and be supportively present to her children and grandchildren. The caregiver must have the ability to listen and have the patience to let her talk about her past, and then use every opportunity that offers an opening to reassure her self-worth and self-confidence. Her strong nurturing capacities that partly arose from her own need to be nurtured emphasize her present needs. They can now be turned into a new strength for self-acceptance and for reaching out to others. Her own psychological structure is simultaneously her weakness and her strength, and plays a central role in the grieving and healing process.

Similar dynamics are involved in the struggle of John, a priest in his mid-fifties. He had a successful career in teaching and counseling. Later he became pastor of a large parish and held several important functions in the diocese. He was the oldest of three children and the only son in an Italian family, very much loved and revered by his parents and sisters. He was very close to his father. At the height of John's personal success, his father died of cancer. Although the shock was enormous, John seemed to take it remarkably well. Grief did not seem to influence his daily activity or priestly ministry.

Shortly after his father's death, however, an earlier ear problem began to act up and led to ear surgery for John. Bronchitis began to plague him and did not go away. Several weeks of complete rest in a warmer climate did not help. His condition grew worse and tests showed that cancer had developed in his colon and metastasized in his liver, lungs, and pancreas. The diagnosis was devastating, and the prognosis was very poor.

No one can prove that the lack of appropriate grieving for his father's death caused or even contributed to John's illness and cancer. His cancer was very real and very physical, and could not be reduced to a case of deep depression. We know, however, that grief for the loss of a loved one can seriously undermine human resistance to illness and opens the way for malignancies. John was also a person who needed to play center stage, but his illness made that impossible. This was another trauma that may have contributed to the weakening of his immune system.

To minister effectively to John, his emotional well-being needs to be taken into account. He needs continuously to increase his awareness of the independent value of his own life. The success of his past ministry and the importance of his present position can be elements in affirming his inner personal value, but they do not form the basic value of his life. They are not proof of his importance. They are only an affirmation of his talents and the effective ways in which he utilizes them. John needs to deepen his sense of his personal value independent from his position of importance, which, in fact, he did magnificently. His courage did not cure his cancer, but it did help him to find deeper personal value and wholeness in his own life, even in the midst of apparent physical disintegration. With this sense of personal wholeness his illness took on a different meaning.

Growing Through Pain and Suffering

If life is equated with success in one's job, then illness is an enemy that fights against the meaning of life. If life is a search for personal wholeness that strives for a balance among the material, psychological, and spiritual perspectives of human existence, then illness is part of the outline that describes the conditions in which this balance of wholeness is to be achieved. The structure of the personality plays an important role in the healing (or integrative) process of the one who suffers.

The foregoing reflections suggest that the emotional depth of grief is a cause of deep personal pain that can contribute to physical ailments, but it can also be part of the healing process. A detailed discussion on grief is not appropriate or possible at this point. It must be emphasized, however, that the structure of the personality is an important determinant in the way grief affects an individual and in the way the individual responds to his or her new condition.

Emotional pain which is not the result of a loss, but which comes forth from the structure of the personality itself is another form of suffering. Although this book is not geared toward the mental health aspect of healthcare ministry, it cannot completely pass over this topic in silence. Even if a person seems to be functioning effectively, emotional pain can place an extraordinary burden on an individual and contribute to physical inability. If such a person indeed falls ill, the handling of the illness will be deeply interwoven with his or her psychological condition. The experience of Helen may help to clarify this.

As a child, Helen was sexually abused by her grandfather and uncle for an extended period of time. Helen felt that she had no way of resisting, nor could she speak about it with anyone in the family. Threats by the abusers filled her with fear, and the abusers' status in the family convinced her that no one would ever believe her. She carried the burden alone and felt increasingly unworthy, indecent, and valueless. She did reasonably well in school and secured a good job. Although she had no suicidal tendencies, life had no attraction for her. Normal illnesses like colds and flu gave her more problems than one might expect in an otherwise healthy person. When she fell seriously ill with pneumonia, she seemed to have no strength to fight the fever and the infections connected with it. No physical reason could be pinpointed, but she had no zest for life.

With the help of a competent chaplain, Helen began to take a serious look at herself. In a slow process of encouragement and reflection, she began to see how her self-evaluation was tainted by her childhood experiences. She began to understand that what had happened to her did not diminish the value of her personality or the decency of her being. She learned to accept the fact that her personal value was not destroyed, but was masked by the indecency of others. Slowly she returned to full physical health and to a psychological wholeness which she had never before known. There is no doubt that Helen's illness was physical, but the way she coped with her illness had a strong psychological basis.

The few examples in this chapter only scratch the surface. They are intended to demonstrate how illness and suffering, or rather how the manner in which illness and suffering are approached, correspond to the structure of the personality. This does not mean that only a counselor or therapist can effectively deal with patients. Far from it. Most patients have the inner strength to cope with both physical and emotional problems, but the understanding presence of a friend or minister can be invaluable.

Each of the examples in this chapter demonstrates the chapter title by pointing out the path of suffering from disintegration to growth. Joe and James in their accidents, Elly in her bereavement, John in his bereavement and illness, and Helen in her emotional pain show us that the life they had built was disintegrating. The very disintegrating factor, however, became the challenge and the opportunity to reconstruct their lives and develop areas of strength that were untapped resources deep within them.

No one wants to suffer, but no one can avoid it. For those who can handle it, the seemingly destructive forces of suffering can be turned into significant opportunities for human wholeness.

Notes

1. Joseph Fichter, *Religion and Pain* (New York: Crossroad, 1981), p. 18.

2. van der Poel, *The Integration of Human Values*, pp. 93-94.

3. Cornelius J. van der Poel, *Health Care Ministry and the Meaning of Human Suffering*, unpublished manuscript, Barry University 1993 pp. 55 ff.

Chapter Six

Suffering—A Religious Experience

Suffering is inseparable from the human reality, so much so that it is part of the essence of being human. Human life without suffering is unthinkable. In fact, human life without suffering cannot be fully human in the world as we know it. History shows that no period of human existence has been without suffering, yet no one has ever presented a satisfactory explanation for the presence and reality of suffering.

Suffering is a mystery that escapes human understanding. One of the basic reasons for the mysterious nature of suffering may lie in the insight that "suffering is not a theoretical problem which reasoning can resolve. Pain can never be merely under*stood*; it is a situation which can only be under*gone*, through human (Christian) believing Praxis."[1]

Suffering as Integral to the Human Condition

This statement implies that suffering is beyond human understanding and has something to do with the human relationship with God. If we accept two basic assumptions: (1) that the human being is created by God, and (2) that history indicates that humanity never existed (cannot exist) without suffering, then we must accept some form of relationship between creation and suffering. Teilhard de Chardin, the late Jesuit paleontologist and theologian, considers suffering "a necessary by-product of evolution."[2]

In the created cosmos, development includes a transition from one stage to another. We experience some form of suffering (insecurity) when we let go of familiar surroundings and venture into the unknown. This occurs, for instance, when we move to a new place or start a new job. It also happens as we move through developmental phases in our lives.

In previous chapters we have discussed the pain that can occur in one's transition from childhood to maturity. Every step toward maturity has its own worries and insecurities. We usually do not call such transitions suffering, but in the final analysis they are. We see this more clearly when our strength declines, when we feel that we are disintegrating, or when we approach the ultimate human disintegration of death.

Johanna's struggle to accept her final illness and face the reality of her own death offers an example of the painfulness of this transition. She had lived a full life, but not without pain. As a young woman she wanted to become a nun. She entered a convent, but during the novitiate she developed tuberculosis and could not continue. She went back to her parents for rest and cure. After she was cured her parents needed her at home. In time she married and raised a family. At age seventy she developed breast cancer which later metastasized in her bones. Her physician managed to keep her pain under control so that she could continue to live a relatively active life. Chemotherapy slowed down the progress of cancer but step by step she saw her life ebbing away. Still there was no complaint. She viewed each new day as a gift from God. Her motto became, "The best I can do is all I can do, and I will leave the rest to God." As long as medication could help her live she would continue. How different this attitude is from that of the advocates of assisted suicide who prefer to hasten death rather than to accept the challenge of living one's life the best one can in all circumstances.

These disintegrating experiences are beyond human control, although their occurrence and their form can be modified by human intervention. Personality development is an important factor in the way individuals approach suffering and deal with it. Human decision making is significantly influenced by the way an individual either copes with or avoids suffering.

Suffering is part of the fabric of human life. It forces individuals and the community to acknowledge their own limitations. Where human desires and dreams aim for perfection, flawlessness, and unlimited satisfaction, daily life repeatedly presents situations that go beyond human strength and understanding.

Turning to Religion for Meaning

Faced with their inability to control their own health or their surroundings, people often turn to religion. J. Milton Yinger (as quoted by Joseph Fichter) explains that when people turn to religion in the face of suffering,

> they express their refusal to capitulate to death, to give up in the face of frustration, and to allow hostility to tear apart their human associations. The quality of being religious, seen from the individual's point of view, implies two things: first, a belief that evil, pain, bewilderment, and injustice are fundamental facts of existence; and second, a set of practices and related sanctified beliefs that express a conviction that man [sic] can ultimately be saved from these facts.[3]

Turning to religion involves a human effort to search for a central meaning in life despite regular experiences of pain and frustration. When life has meaning, people experience a special strength that motivates and enables them to cope with problems more effectively. Throughout his book, *Man's Search for Meaning,* Victor Frankl points out that people with deep religious faith had a significantly greater chance to survive the cruelty of concentration camps than those whose lives had lost all meaning. Greshake puts it this way:

> Where there is no suffering, the earnestness, depth and dignity which characterize maturity may also be lacking. If a person refuses to confront the contrary and awkward side of reality, but rather seeks to evade every uncomfortable situation, and takes refuge in a self-constructed, fortified "healthy world," then he or she remains infantile, immature, faceless.[4]

The effective handling of suffering is an important factor in growth toward maturity and productivity in human life. Times of disaster and great human need are frequently also times of invention and creativity. The same holds true for times of emotional, psychological, and spiritual hardship. These are the times we can expect the most radical (trans-)formation of the personality, the times in which understanding, sensitivity, and compassion will develop. Suffering becomes productive only when the individual does not strike back at it, but utilizes his or her condition of suffering as an opportunity for growth.

Learning to Cope with Suffering and Grief

Coping with crises involves a learning process. At first glance suffering seems contrary to human nature, but once one can integrate it into one's personal approach to life, a higher degree of maturity can be reached than would otherwise be possible.

My own Aunt Nelly, who died some fifty years ago, is a perfect example of someone who learned to cope with suffering. For approximately twenty years of her relatively short life she was in and out of hospitals and sanatoriums suffering from an incurable form of tuberculosis. Most of her days were spent between bed and chair. She could do no physical work, although she did an unbelievable amount of needlepoint and crocheting. What she did best of all and most of all, however, was to be the confidante of everyone else in the family. Her own limitations and suffering had become the vehicle for her to develop a deep sense of concern and understanding for others. Her illness never got her down and she proved a support for anyone who had difficulty dealing with life. Aunt Nelly saw her illness as part of life. She not only did not complain about it, but conveyed God's love by helping others in the best way she could. Her illness was the vehicle for personal and religious growth.

Erika Schuchardt, utilizing the stages of grief developed by Elisabeth Kübler-Ross, describes a learning process that leads to internal freedom and maturity.[5] She describes how this growth process takes place in three stages of knowing, experiencing/feeling, and realizing.

The initial stage is the *cognitive stage.* It is characterized by questions that start with *Uncertainty* (What is really going on?), and lead to *Certainty* (Yes, it did happen), mixed with *Denial* (But it still can't be true). This stage projects a cognitive dimension which stays at an external level.

The second stage is the *transit stage.* It is characterized by strong emotions of *Aggression* (Why me?), of *Negotiation* (But if..., then...), and *Depression* (What for? It's all pointless...). In this stage the internalization process begins to take place, and focuses on the person's emotional experience. Reality is recognized (Stage One), but it is rejected at an emotional level (Stage Two). The individual who is suffering does not yet allow the loss, pain, or grief to become an influential factor in his or her life.

Finally there is the *target stage*, which is characterized by action. Starting with *Acceptance* (Now I begin to realize...), this stage expresses itself first in a self-assured *Activity* (I'll handle it!), which is eventually modified to *Solidarity* (We're handling it together!). Through this solidarity the suffering individual experiences a new self-value as he or she reaches out to friends and to the community, and develops a new self-image that is stronger and more mature than before.

This learning process, as presented by Schuchardt, centers around a change of attitude. The individual journeys from a denial of reality via a process of recognition to an integrated wholeness. The individual does not seek suffering or love it when it does occur, but allows it to become a constituent in his or her self-realization. The individual's attitude changes in the face of the inescapable reality of pain and suffering. From this perspective Richard Vieth points out: "Because religion is a basic shaper of attitudes and dispositions, faith will profoundly inform the way we perceive and respond to affliction."[6]

Changing Perceptions About God

In *The Search for Human Values*, I argued that God is understood according to the human ability of perception.[7] Education, culture, life experience, and personality all play a role in how an individual understands God. Innumerable times we have heard sick people say, "It is God's will," or "God is testing me," or "Why does God punish me?" In the mind of many people all suffering comes from God. Whether they question God's love and justice, accept God's decision blindly, or curse God for the illness they suffer, they acknowledge a relationship between God and pain. They also acknowledge that the pain they suffer is an important factor in their attitude toward God, whether this attitude is marked by anger or love. Suffering is an important factor in how all people—both those who suffer and those who minister to them in their suffering—shape and express their religious convictions.

A person's religious outlook on life is ultimately a free choice on the part of the individual. Education and the early formation of the personality can exercise a great influence on one's religious beliefs, but in the final analysis, it is the individual who takes responsibility for his or her own religious convictions. An individual has to decide to accept suffering and integrate it into his or her religious perspective if the person is to benefit from suffering and grow because of it.

Greshake points out that God absolutely does not will suffering.[8] What God wills is the growth process of each individual. Greshake focuses on how God's power and love lie at the center of all existence, including human existence. Having created humankind with the task of growing into full selfhood by integrating the finite with the infinite, the material with the spiritual, God's presence lies at the heart of the human growth process and, therefore, also at the core of human suffering. Whenever the growth process includes suffering, we may say that God's presence lies at the heart of human suffering. This presence "issues in God sharing in the very suffering of man [sic], so that he [sic] enables the person to overcome it as it is. This means that God himself [sic] enters into the suffering of humanity."[9] By entering into human suffering God does not take over from people, but rather enables them to live their lives with all their human qualities within the limits which their condition allows.

The teaching and life of Jesus amply indicate that Christianity does not free people from suffering. On the contrary, Jesus makes it very clear that anyone who wants to be his disciple must take up his or her own cross and follow Jesus. At no point, however, does Jesus indicate that his disciples should seek suffering. They don't have to look for suffering; suffering will present itself to them.

The presence of God will be experienced amid people's suffering and pain in accordance with the nature and structure of their individual personalities. Anxious, self-rejecting people will be strongly inclined to experience the punishing and rejecting presence of God. Suffering is likely to increase their anxiety and lower their self-image. Reassuring them of God's goodness and justice will give them little support.

Self-accepting people will have an easier time integrating suffering into the fabric of their lives and seeing it as a new challenge, and not as a divine punishment. They will also be more likely in their search for health to see suffering as part of the circumstances within which they are called to realize their total self.

Suffering, indeed, is a major factor in the process of growth and wholeness. It is also a major force toward holiness, since the experience of inescapable dependence is an invitation to surrender to God. St. Paul expresses this when he writes: "When I experience my weakness, it is then that I am strong" (2 Cor 12:10). In illness, faith can step beyond a reliance on the human so that people can surrender themselves into the loving arms of the Creator.

Notes

1. Gisbert Greshake. "Human Suffering and the Question of God," *Stauros Bulletin*, 1 (1977), p. 5.
2. Greshake, *op. cit.*, p. 30.
3. Fichter, *Religion and Pain*, p. 20.
4. Greshake, *op. cit.*, p. 26.

5. Erika Schuchardt, *Why Is this Happening to Me? Guidance and Hope for Those Who Suffer* (Minneapolis: Augsburg Fortress, 1989), pp. 24-42.

6. Richard F. Vieth, *Holy Power, Human Pain* (New York: Meyer Stone Books, 1988), p. 13.

7. van der Poel, *The Search for Human Values,* pp. 16-20.

8. Greshake, *op. cit.,* p. 33.

9. Greshake, *op. cit.,* p. 34.

Chapter Seven

Suffering — Gateway to Wholeness

If suffering is an unavoidable reality in human life, then it is also an unavoidable and indispensable element in human self-realization. Nobody likes suffering and we all make every possible effort to overcome it and eliminate it, but we cannot live our human lives without seriously taking the reality of suffering into account.

Taking this position involves accepting a number of assumptions. The most important of these is that humankind is created in the image of God. This image is not based on a similarity of features, actions, or tone of voice. It is a sharing in being. God's being is spiritual and infinite. It cannot be contained or adequately manifested in material or finite ways, yet the humans who share in God's being have the task of giving expression to this spiritual reality in daily human life.

Spiritual perspectives form an essential dimension of human wholeness. To see human life exclusively in material and psychological dimensions shortchanges the wholeness of both individuals and the community. On the other hand, to focus exclusively on the spiritual values of human existence and act as if material aspects are only a sort of prison in which the human spirit is temporarily contained, equally violates human dignity and wholeness. The balance lies in a process of integration that gives full respect and credit to the material, psychological, and spiritual dimensions simultaneously.

Material existence is individualistic by nature and turns inward for self-preservation and continuation. Psychological dimensions do not exist on their own, but are alive and operative in certain forms of material existence. They have the ability to find completeness and strength by reaching beyond the material, self-oriented world to a level of conscious receiving and self-giving. A person's psychological consciousness animates and gives meaning to individual existence and causes the person to reach beyond himself or herself and give a wider meaning to creation. A person's psychological dimension does not elevate material existence beyond itself, but helps the person to break through individualism and isolation.

A person's spiritual inclinations also do not exist on their own in the human reality. They are inseparably connected with a form of individualization in which the spiritual dimension is integrated with the material and psychological reality of human life. Its task (or its nature or being) is to communicate to the material and psychological dimensions a perspective and meaning that reach beyond the self-oriented striving of material existence. The spiritual dimension elevates a person beyond material and individualistic values into a realm of different values and realities. This elevation is the origin of an integration which constitutes the wholeness of human life. Through this integration the life of God is shared with human beings and is manifested in the limitations of created existence.

This blending of the spiritual with the material and psychological aspects of human life imposes certain restrictions on the material and psychological perspectives. The material must let go of that individualism which turns it exclusively toward itself. The psychological must allow itself to be called into a realm beyond that of individualistic self-realization. The spiritual needs to clothe its quest for infinity in the finiteness of created and perceptible existence.

This process of integration brings us face to face with a being that is wholly present in the material cosmic reality, yet above which it rises through an experience of being that reaches into the realm of the divine. This straddling of the material and spiritual is a wondrous and inexplicable mystery, but it also creates a built-in and unavoidable source of tension and human suffering.

The Challenge of Personal Integration

Human wholeness is found in the integration of the material, psychological, and spiritual dimensions of a person's being. This three-way integration cannot take place without suffering. Earlier chapters discussed the interaction between the material and psychological-emotional perspectives, and the way they complement and influence each other. The next important question is how the spiritual dimension of human existence influences human wholeness.

While spiritual dimensions do not result from any activity of material or psychological qualities, spiritual dimensions express themselves necessarily in and through a person's material and psychological qualities. While the grace of God can never be produced by human power, it will be present in a person in the shape and form of that individual's personal qualities. Saints Maria Goretti and Thomas Aquinas were each driven by deep faith in God and by an unconditional love for God. Yet this faith and love took on very different forms in the simple little girl and the highly skilled scholar. This difference was not only a result of the circumstances of their lives (where and when they lived, etc.), but also because of the differences in their personalities through which they expressed their faith. God's being and God's strength were the same for both, yet God's presence was, as it were, adapted to each individual. God animated each of them in such a way that they both reached their full potential by using the talents God gave them.

This insight might help us to understand better the role of spiritual values in the experience of human suffering. God's presence (the spiritual values in human existence) is recognized according to the individual's personality, and in turn, it shapes the personality. Reflection on the way the Christian virtues of faith, hope, and love are expressed and shaped by the human person may help us to see what this means.

The Power of Faith

Faith is considered to be one of the divine (supernatural) virtues because the content of faith falls, by its nature, outside the realm of human abilities and understanding. Faith is the (often unconscious) acceptance and awareness of one's dependence on a power beyond one's control. Many different names can be given to this power. We may call it God, fate, or a similar name. In its deepest reality, however, faith is the human recognition that we are dependent on a power beyond our control. One may acknowledge this dependence or deny it, submit to it or fight it, collaborate with it or drag one's feet. In the final analysis these are all forms of recognition, and each of these responses shapes our human response to that power.

The awareness of this power within us awakens in two major steps. First, there is a message that comes from the outside, either by words or by experience: We are told about God by parents or elders, or we experience our own limitations. This external message, however, will have no effect unless it corresponds to an internal experience. Jesuit theologian Karl Rahner states:

Faith is never awakened by someone having something communicated to a person purely from the outside, addressed solely to the naked understanding as such. To lead to faith (or rather to its further explicit stage) is always to assist understanding of what has already been experienced in the depth of human reality as grace (i.e., as in absolutely direct relation to God).[1]

The message that comes from outside confirms the vague and undetermined awareness that arises from the depth of human reality. It leads to a reaction with which the individual feels at ease and which leads to specific forms of self-expression.

Faith is a form of self-realization. The individual personality expresses itself *vis-à-vis* a power that is beyond its own control, but which is experienced as an essential dimension of one's being. In some ways this dynamic is similar to the first of Erikson's stages (Basic Trust vs. Basic Mistrust). Integrating the physical (material), psychological, and spiritual dimensions of one's being leads to a most basic self-realization or underlying self-image. This self-image is the vision of one's personal value. Full acceptance by others leads to trust, while rejection by others leads to mistrust. One of the significant "others" who enables a person to experience trust (or mistrust) is God.

Dependence on a power beyond one's control is marked by these same categories. If one has experienced loving acceptance in the early stages of total dependence, the ultimate power is also easily seen as an accepting and loving power with whom it is easy to collaborate. The early experience of mistrust, caused by a lack of acceptance and love, predisposes the person to a suspicious attitude. One has to guard oneself against an ultimate power that adopts those characteristics. The difference between these extremes is seen quite often in daily life.

For some people God is a loving parent; for others, God is a fearsome, punitive authority. Accordingly, whatever happens in the life of a trusting person will be experienced as a sign of love, as a challenge to grow, and as a call to respond with greater love. The mistrusting person is likely to see all happenings either as a reward or a punishment from God based on what he or she has or has not done. When people find their deepest personal value in external acceptance and affirmation rather than in the depths of their being, the same can be expected of their relationship with God.

In his book, *Religion and Pain,* Joseph Fichter points to three different religious reactions that people have toward illness.[2] First, there are those who are totally absorbed in secularism. They may live a life of politeness and kindness, but they have no need for a personal relationship with God. They simply ignore God. Second, others have a personal relationship and seek divine intervention even though their lives may not be very religious overall. For some of these people, God is at the center of their lives, but more often God is a power that is supposed to provide what they want or need, rather than a source of life and growth. Finally, there are those who deny God's existence. They are or become atheists.

Anyone who is in frequent contact with sick people has met all three categories. To those who seem not to need God, one can be a significant support on the mere psychological level by conveying respect and acceptance. In those who deny God, one has a good chance to encounter hostility. Discussions about God are often useless. The best help one can give to such persons is frequently limited to showing concern and interest in their condition. Whatever defensiveness or emptiness there may be within them usually cannot be resolved at this stage of their lives. Unless there are indications that suggest otherwise, it is usually better not to disturb their (relative) peace of mind when death is approaching, particularly when they seem to be persons of honesty and sincerity. If they recover from their illness, the experience of understanding and kindness will open more doors to faith than will intellectual discussions.

Faith plays a different role in the lives of people who accept God's power. The chaplain will find, however, that their faith often needs to be purified and to grow. Most people who work in pastoral ministry have heard innumerable times: "I don't deserve this. Why is God punishing me?" Underneath this expression of surprise or discontent lies a personality trait that is deeply concerned about the acceptable results of their activities. They see good health as a reward for obedience, good works, and observance of the law. Illness is the opposite; it is the punishment for disobedience, sin, and breaking of the law. Such a relationship with God is established by being most concerned about the letter of the law. A common result is mistrust, bitterness, and depression. Without trying to pigeon-hole anyone, such persons seem to fall under the second category described by Fichter: God has an importance in their life, but God is seen more as a paymaster than as a source of life.

Joe's acceptance of Mary's death and his involvement in the arrangements for her funeral are an amazing display of strength and balance in his personality (see pages 46-48). His deep faith was a very significant part of his personality. His inner strength and sense of personal worth were not merely a psychological development. He was strengthened and found his wholeness and integration in his relationship with God. His relationship with God was not so much a servile attitude, but rather an experience of union and love. The acceptance of his condition was not a fatalistic acceptance of "this power beyond his reach from which he could not escape." Joe accepted the presence of

God as a constant invitation to collaborate with others in expressing love, compassion, and respect at the death of his wife. His faith did not lead to numbness or insensitivity. It was a source of wholeness that enabled him to extend his active love for Mary beyond her physical life and to plan her funeral liturgy with his children, with whom he felt united in an unbreakable bond of love. For Joe, faith was a life-giving power that made him more deeply human, united him with others, and transformed his human capacities to a level beyond their own reach.

The case of James and Sue shows a slightly different approach (pages 17-19 and pages 48-49). There is no doubt that God played a role in James' life, but God *owed* him a few things. James had been faithful in his duties toward God; he had used his talents effectively, and cared for his wife and children. He had *proven* himself a person of value, so why did this accident happen to him? James felt that his goodness and acceptability were destroyed in the accident, and because of this God made it impossible for him to express properly his love for his wife and children. James' knowledge of God was focused upon the *rewarding* (or punishing) God.

James had to rediscover his own value as a person before he could discover the love of God. In this process of rediscovery the insight of full acceptability before God, even with a physical handicap, was a powerful means in his search for wholeness. He was able to blend spiritual and psychological values into the oneness of an acceptable personality. God, the *authority* in James' life, also became the source of love and value. When he was healthy, James had been able to cover up his insecurity. His handicap revealed the brokenness of the inner person, but it also became the bridge that effectively straddled the gap between the material and spiritual aspects of his personality. His relationship with God became the power that healed the wound of brokenness that was ripped open by his accident.

Many other factors are involved in developing and maintaining a healthy adult personality. Just as self-acceptance lies at the base of a healthy personality, so faith lies at the foundation of the human relationship with God. But faith alone cannot maintain this relationship. Other human attitudes are necessary to complete the basis for this relationship, namely hope and love.

The Importance of Hope

Hope is the human attitude by which people are aware of their limitations but simultaneously expect that by applying their abilities, they can achieve all or a significant part of their goals. This human attitude can be related to the early stage in life where children begin to explore by crawling, standing, walking, grabbing, and touching. The experience of limitations does not hold children back from trying to satisfy insatiable curiosity. The loving assistance and wise guidance of adults help children develop their autonomy and minimize the shame and doubt caused by failure.

Based upon this encouragement, a child learns to commit him or herself and to reach out trustingly. This is the beginning of love. The child has experienced himself or herself as an acceptable person, and has the ability to let go of defensiveness and be open to others even when life gets rough.

The Christian virtue of hope expresses itself in and through human qualities. When the goods at which we aim seem to be out of reach, it is trust in our own qualities and in the goodness and reliability of others that keeps us going. A genuine trust in God cannot be brought forth by mere human efforts, but God's gift of hope can be blended with human capacities to give a special strength to all human efforts.

Too often in situations of suffering, pain, illness, and injury, we confuse hope with the human desire to regain physical health. Its real strength and meaning become manifest in the readiness to do whatever our capacities allow us to do. With the insight that God calls us not necessarily to physical health but to human wholeness, hope becomes the power that prevents discouragement. A material object such as physical health may be beyond human reach, but the ability to activate one's present talents within the circumstances of life can always be achieved. This hope never dies.

In certain circumstances we see hope unfolding in subsequent stages, as in the case of a patient who initially hopes to be cured completely from cancer. When that does not work, the hope is set on arresting it for some years. Finally, all he or she asks for is the opportunity to make the best of the remaining days or hours. Hope is the ability to adapt and to utilize one's limited powers.

In daily life it is impossible to point out where the human quality of hope stops and the virtue starts. For the believing person, they blend together at every moment and in all circumstances. In the case of James and Sue, hope played an important role. James had to learn to accept himself as a one-armed engineer, but before he could do that he had to trust that others could accept him in that way. His faith in God's acceptance nudged him gently in that direction.

The Necessity of Love

Hope can be activated only if a person has the courage to reach out for what he or she wants to achieve. Love is active self-fulfillment utilizing all the qualities and talents that one has. It presupposes self-acceptance and trust in the person who loves. Love finds its fulfillment in being accepted by (or being united with) the object of one's love. In a person's search for health, it is love that helps the patient accept him or herself at every moment and in every condition. Love provides the strength to make the best of life without anger or bitterness.

To the extent that a person's being is permeated by the strength of faith and hope, there is a ground for the virtue of love. The virtue of love in its purest form—as a love for God in one's life—becomes a major factor in the search for healing and wholeness. The experience of Joe and his ability to become actively involved in his wife's funeral and his own recovery, despite his wife's death, was greatly inspired by his love for God. There was a wholeness in his personality that could not be defeated by sorrow or pain. Self-activation remained a major perspective in his life. This included reaching out to others in such a way that by reaching out to others he reached out to God.

These few examples and applications provide a general idea of how a person reacts to illness and how religion plays a significant role in the pursuit of recovery and wholeness. It is the task of the pastoral worker or caregiver to be sensitive not only to the needs of those who suffer, but also to the potentialities of their personality and talents.

Chapter Nine will consider how further developmental stages contribute in their own way to the human response to suffering. The next chapter will address the impact of the suffering of one family member on his or her family, and on the others who lives are impacted by the suffering.

Notes

1. Karl Rahner, "Faith" in *Encyclopedia of Theology: The Concise Sacramentum Mundi* (New York: Seabury, 1975), p. 497.
2. Fichter, *Religion and Pain*, pp. 55-64.

Chapter Eight

How Suffering Affects a Family

Suffering has far-reaching effects. Just as the life of each individual affects the lives of many others, so the suffering of one person influences the lives of others. Since an individual does not exist and cannot live in total isolation, he or she will not respond to the circumstances of life in a totally isolated manner.

The development and maintenance of one's personality are inextricably interwoven with human interaction. The early human growth process is a clear example of this. The newborn is completely powerless and dependent. The child's only means of survival is to rely on the protection of others and to adapt to their demands. This need for adaptation becomes so ingrained that it largely determines the shape of an individual's personality. According to individual necessities, this need can lead to any form of behavior from fearful suspicion and defensiveness to loving and spontaneous collaboration.

Family life and familial relationships lie at the center of this development. Family members display a need for interdependence which is considerably stronger than most other intimate relationships. The lasting effects of parental influence on early childhood development are, at least in theory, widely known and recognized. To understand the manner in which a person reacts to the demands of life, therefore, it is important to be acquainted with the person's background and origins. To heal a disharmony in a person one needs to know with whom this individual must harmonize and what are the characteristics of the other members of the family.

These general statements are quite important for understanding all forms of human suffering, including emotional suffering. For example, overbearing parental authority is confining and demeaning, and can create a feeling of unworthiness in the developing person. Such feelings are a source of emotional suffering which, at some point in life, may become too much for the individual to carry. It could even lead to a breakdown for which the person will need professional assistance. The effects of parental and sibling influence are not restricted to emotional development. They have an impact upon the individual's response to physical illness as well.

The illness of one member often changes many things in the life of a family. The usual routine is broken. Specific tasks remain undone, or other family members must substitute for the sick one, usually over and above their own responsibilities. The atmosphere of the family relationship changes when one person needs special care for an extended period of time. When the illness is not very serious, or when it lasts only a short period of time, there is usually no problem. Most people consider it a privilege to care for a loved one for a few days. This caring does not ask for much adjustment. Greater adaptation is required if an illness is prolonged and disabling, because then relationships may change and adjustments will be more radical. These conditions cause a form of suffering in the healthy as well as in the sick.

It is impossible to study in detail all the various human relationships that are affected by the sickness of an individual. I will restrict myself to the impact of illness upon the family and to the impact that the family's reaction has upon the sick person.

The Role of the Family
in the Development of the Personality

A family is not a group of people who come together by accident or by chance. The family constitutes a bond that is created by a personal choice and decision. The nature of the choice, however, leaves its mark on the nature of the bond itself. If a deep and mature love lies at the origin of this bond, the relationship will be characterized by creative reaching out to each other in mutual complementarity. They will also reach beyond themselves in a life-giving, creative activity.

Sometimes, however, the family bond arises from the needs of lonely individuals who seek reassurance of their own value by attaching themselves to others. This was discussed earlier in the sixth psychosocial crisis (Intimacy vs. Isolation).

Sometimes marriages begin out of a felt need to legitimize a child whose conception was not intended, with no thought of developing the relationship between husband and wife. Circumstances like these influence the nature of the family bond and the personality of the children.

Despite this variety of circumstances there are certain characteristics that are common to most family relationships, and the way they influence the human response to suffering. This chapter will consider several different family structures and analyze the impact they have on people's reactions to suffering and pain.

Family bonds arise from a conscious decision of the partners, whether this decision be motivated by genuine love, passion, anger, personal insecurity, or some other dynamic. The bond that is a result of genuine love will create a different atmosphere than will the bond that arises when a marriage is entered into for personal security or financial profit. In a healthy, happy marriage, the sickness of one of the partners will not easily create alienation. The partner who is ill will not be made to feel that he or she is a burden to the relationship. The constant experience of love and acceptance, even in a time of illness, is a support for the patient as well as for the healthy partner. However painful the illness may be for the healthy partner, genuine love will strengthen the couple as they carry their heavy load together.

When the basis of the bond is insecurity, anger, or profit, the relationship will be affected differently. If the marriage was born out of immature or improper motives, the illness of one partner may cause the healthy partner to experience a form of betrayal. If the bond was begun as a form of self-protection, illness attacks the very reason for the existence of the marriage. The sick person becomes a burden which either takes away the profit, increases the anger, or destroys the security. Such a relationship undermines the self-esteem of the sick person and causes a special form of suffering for the marriage partner.

The example of James and Sue shows how their relationship went through a radical change after James' accident (pages 17-19). It was not only James who suffered; his wife faced hard times as well. At the basis of this suffering lies the structure of their personalities, in particular James' need to prove himself. If this and similar couples are to be helped, the caregiver must have an awareness of the inter-relationship of the couple.

The relationship between the marriage partners has repercussions on the children. The initial total dependence of the children on their parents creates an almost unbreakable attachment on the part of the children. Even in adolescence, when teenagers may seem to rebel against parental authority, the inexplicable yearning for acceptance remains.

The shape and nature of the relationship between the parents has a direct influence on the parent-child relationship. A loving and trusting relationship between the parents is likely to convey this trust to the children, and build personalities that are trusting and able to reach out. Such children do not have to prove anything. If the child becomes ill, there is less danger for feelings of rejection or lack of value. The impact of a child's illness upon his or her parents will be less destructive when a relationship is based upon love. Their dreams and goals are less involved with profit or external appearance and more concerned about life and happiness.

Earlier we discussed how faith and religious values are shaped by the structure of the personality. Family structures are important shapers of children's faith and color their outlook toward suffering and pain. Faith, it must be recalled, is a form of trusting and surrender; it includes a feeling of acceptance and personal importance. For the trusting person, God is more than a supplier of life and all material things connected with it. For such a person, God is the basic source of life, who challenges individuals to respond to what life offers. Illness, then, is not experienced as a punishment either by the parents or by the child. Illness challenges them to use all available human resources, but their desire for a total return to physical health is modified by their concern to give the best human response they can. They may not say this in so many words, but their acceptance of situations as they occur, and their peace of mind in all circumstances, speak more eloquently than words. The mutual interdependence and trust between parents and children is either strengthened or weakened through illness. It will never stay the same.

In cases of illness the family bond often takes on a different shape and urgency. When a partner in marriage is ill, a new, unexpected, and sometimes heavy burden is placed on the healthy partner. This is usually very easy for a short period of time, but in the long run it can become very difficult if not unbearable. If the "housekeeper" is disabled, other solutions must be found. If the "breadwinner" is put out of action, the family may have to prepare for hard times. Personality structures determine largely how the sick person can handle "being cared for." The attitude of the sick person has a great influence on the response of the healthy person to the increased responsibilities.

Michael and Mary were not the happiest couple. He was a good provider, but impatient, violent, and given to drinking. Particularly on weekends Michael was unapproachable and unbearable. His family of origin had given him the message that the wife's role in marriage was housework and service. Mary was sickly and needed support and tender care which Michael could not give, and which he did not intend to try to give. The oldest son had to take over much of the care that the father did not provide. Running errands, helping around the house, taking care of the younger children, and many other chores fell to him. In addition, he was also his mother's confidant and had to listen, even as a young child, to her tales of woe about how his father maltreated her. Often he heard stories that were far beyond his comprehension.

In this case, the mother's illness was not only a reason for frustration on the part of the husband; it also prevented the little boy from behaving and thinking as a child. He carried with him all the consequences of such a situation. These consequences became evident when he became an adult and was torn between the need to help others and the resentment of helping others, which he experienced as being imposed upon. This often resulted in unreasonable outbursts of anger. A long and painful healing process was necessary to repair this early damage.

The Impact of Illness on Family Relationships

Since family relationships contribute greatly to shape the personalities of family members, the illness of one family member significantly affects the emotions, behavior, and growth process of other family members. This was evident in the relationship between Michael and Mary and in the consequences for their oldest son. The illness of the parent had profound repercussions on the children. While the illness of a parent is usually more disruptive to the growth process of the family, a child's illness can also have serious consequences for the whole family.

This is illustrated in the life of Arthur and Anne, two middle-class professionals. He was an engineer, she was a teacher. They had four children ranging in age from eight to fifteen. The oldest fell sick and, after a long period of testing, was diagnosed as having an inoperable brain tumor. The location and nature of the tumor affected his respiratory system so much that he had to be kept alive by a respirator. Since hospital costs became prohibitive, arrangements were made to have the respirator brought home. Anne was trained to give this care under the daily supervision of a respiratory therapist from a nearby hospital.

Under these circumstances, Edward literally became the center of the family. His bed was located at a spot between the living room and the dining room so that it would be visible from almost every corner of the house. A bulky respirator was next to the bed, and the sounds of its hissing and sucking were audible everywhere. The parents' bedroom door was kept open day and night to make sure that the mother could respond immediately to any irregular sound. Edward's motor abilities were also affected. He had no strength in his arms or legs. He could not sit, walk, hold a book, or feed himself. The otherwise intelligent youth was totally dependent on audio tapes and the people who were willing to read to him.

Edward's share of the household chores was divided among the three younger children. Anne's total involvement with Edward's physical care left many of her chores to the children also. There was little time for the healthy children to play with their friends. They had been used to running and jumping around the house, but that was no longer allowed. Edward could not handle the noise. Their friends who used to walk in and out felt less welcome. When the children came home after school, they were asked to sit with Edward, to tell him about their day, and to read to him. Neither of the parents had much time for the other children since all their activities were centered around Edward. In a word, the children felt that nothing was important but Edward, and although they loved him, they also began to resent him. They felt neglected because of him. Their performance at school deteriorated. They became crabby and their relationship with each other and with their friends became strained.

The happy-go-lucky family did not exist anymore. To aggravate matters even more, Arthur and Anne had no time for each other either. Their social life floundered. Personal intimacies became rare. Minor misunderstandings grew into mutual accusations. Everyday disagreements turned into serious fights. Each member of the family was suffering as a result of one person's serious illness. After a while this kind of home care became too difficult. Edward returned to the hospital, but this gave little relief to the family situation. Anne spent almost all day in the hospital. Arthur visited his son twice a day, and the other children also came on a regular basis. Edward was still very much the center of the family.

This situation may sound extreme, but it is true and gives us an insight into the psychological and emotional problems that can arise from the illness of one family member. The parents could not handle the pressure. Their zeal and generosity were admirable, but an inordinate sense of responsibility prevented them from taking the necessary rest and leaving some care to others. As a result, their relationship suffered serious damage which, in turn, affected the other children. While the children were not toddlers, they still needed the attention of their parents to assure them of their personal value, to show them love, and to let them know that they were as important as Edward. Edward's illness broke down, at least temporarily, much of the initial personality structures that had been built up in their earlier years. When Edward died after a year of suffering, the entire family unit went into counseling.

Evaluating the Effects on the Family

The pastoral minister or caregiver cannot eliminate the effects of illness on the family, but he or she can help families handle themselves appropriately when one of their members is ill. The most basic rule for chaplains is that there is no absolute or pat answer that solves any or all situations. We are always dealing with individuals and individual reactions. There are, however, some general suggestions that may give some direction to the caregiver.

In dealing with any physical illness it is important to know *the importance of bodily integrity for a specific individual.* Age, profession, place in the family, and the degree of dependence on bodily integrity are important factors. The source of self-image and personal value will be another significant influence. A facial disfigurement has a very different meaning for a young woman who is a sales representative than for a man who works in the coal mines. The loss of an arm has a deeper effect on a professional athlete than on an executive who spends most of his or her time in the office. The way that the individual learns to cope with the situation contributes greatly to the way the family will react.

The place of the person in the family unit is another important factor. The sickness of the breadwinner affects the family in a different way than the illness of a retired live-in uncle. The illness of a teenager who is just beginning to try his or her wings will be felt differently than the sickness of an infant. The sick person's place in the family structure affects the demands placed on the coping skills of the family.

Pastoral ministers must also remain alert for the secondary gains that the sick person or any other family member might obtain from the illness. For a person with a poor self-image, a prolonged illness can produce opposing tensions. On the one hand, the illness can deepen the sense of worthlessness, while on the other hand, it can be very attractive to be the center of attention in the family. Manipulative attitudes can flourish in these circumstances.

A third factor is *the patient's attitude toward life*. If social contact is a central element and source of value for a person, then illness threatens the meaning of life. If work is the all-important aspect of life, illness is again a threat to one's very existence. Such patients have the difficult task of changing their lifestyle and value structure, and discontent or anger are likely consequences which will have their impact on the whole family.

If one of the children is ill, other factors come into play. *The importance of the sick child to the parents* plays a significant role. Parents generally love all their children, but each child has his or her own place and significance in the family structure. This has an impact both on how the parents will respond to the sick child, and how they will treat their healthy children.

The age of the sick child in relation to the other children is also important. Younger children need more attention and may feel neglected more easily than older ones. This need may not show immediately, but often it is there. It is not unusual that the effects will manifest themselves at a later age. When Susan, a young adult of twenty-five, had a hard time experiencing herself as a person of value, she often traced these feelings to that time in her childhood when her parents had no time for her. She recalls how they had to take care of Johnnie, her younger brother who was always sick. For some reason that period in her life had left her with a lasting impression of rejection.

It is impossible to discuss all the combinations of circumstances that contribute in their own way to the attitudes and experiences of families who have to deal with serious illness. These few examples should at least alert the chaplain or caregiver to some of the common problems that arise when one member of a family is ill.

The Impact of Family Spirituality on Suffering

Another important question is how a family's spiritual values enter into the process of coping and growth brought about by suffering or illness. There is no simple answer. Keep in mind that religious values are not merely rooted in the individual. Religious values and attitudes originate in the family and flow to the individual.

If a family's faith is primarily characterized by accepting specific points of doctrine and living according to the commandments, there may be little internal religious cohesiveness among the members. They may be bound together by fear or structure, but religious convictions will have little influence on their attitudes towards life. If, however, faith is a lived reality based on the presence of a loving God in human life, religious values will most likely have a much deeper impact on family relationships. In such relationships love and generosity will flourish to a greater depth, mutual acceptance and collaboration will be more spontaneous, and manipulative attitudes will have less chance to develop. In such families, illness can be a source of growth for all. Beautiful human qualities can unfold. Deeply spiritual perspectives can come to the surface, and an unsuspected richness of life can be shared by the family at large.

While this is the briefest of treatments of an important issue from a family perspective, the spiritual perspectives of the human response to suffering considered in Chapter Six offer additional insights to pastors and caregivers, and can be applied to family situations.

Chapter Nine

Suffering and Spiritual Growth

Chapter Five considered some of the general religious values that influence people's reactions to human suffering. Chapter Six focused on the acceptance of suffering as a call or challenge that comes to us from God. This chapter studies the mature way to accept suffering, the manner in which religious values support the human acceptance of suffering, and the way religious values grow and deepen through the acceptance of suffering.

"Maturity" is an elusive term that is used in many different contexts. We can hardly call a ten-year-old boy a mature person, yet I have often stated, both jokingly and seriously, that in a family counseling session a ten-year-old boy may be the only mature person in the group. It is a way of saying that he is the only one who acted according to legitimate expectations regarding age, education, and circumstances. I do not, however, regard the ten-year-old as a mature person.

Maturity is defined as the ability of an adult to assume and carry out responsibilities that correspond to his or her age, education, experience, and position in life. It is entirely possible that an individual who does a wonderful job as a section supervisor in a company, and acts as a very mature person in her position, may not have the maturity to be president of the whole organization. Maturity is a relative term and, although we often consider it as a "present condition," it is more accurately described as a "process" which calls for different perspectives in different circumstances.

The fifth of Erikson's psychosocial stages (Identity vs. Identity Diffusion) is the period in which maturity begins to take shape (see Chapter Four). Bodily organisms and strengths come to full development and intellectual capacities unfold to their fullest extent. The sense and acceptance of one's identity paves the way for more personal relationships with others. It is, however, a period that is characterized by discovery, transition, and adaptation. It can hardly be called a mature age.

Maturity coincides, more or less, with the period of life starting with the sixth psychosocial crisis (Intimacy vs. Isolation). At this stage we expect the individual to be able to share himself or herself with others in a constructive way, so that in the process of sharing both the giver and the receiver grow. They develop their own talents and assist others in developing theirs. They become more deeply themselves, and they become a source of enrichment for others. Although this development hopefully continues in the subsequent stages of Generativity vs. Stagnation and Integrity vs. Despair/Disgust, the stage of Intimacy vs. Isolation is the first stage in which genuine adult maturity may be expected.

The Criteria for Maturity

A mature individual responds appropriately to the various circumstances of life as they occur. At different times and in different circumstances, different responses may be needed. A mature person can make an appropriate judgment, adapt to circumstances, and continue life constructively. Appropriate responses include the individual's responses in times of illness. Gordon Allport states three major criteria for maturity.[1]

1. *The ability to escape immediate biological impulses.*
A mature individual must be able to acknowledge that there are interests and values which go beyond material existence or satisfaction. The mature adult must also be guided by values that come forth from the human psyche (psychogenic), and be concerned with objects and values beyond the range of mere existence-needs (viscerogenic).

Maturity does not exclude concerns about material existence, but is not controlled by them. Think a moment about the relationship between Michael and Mary whom we discussed in the previous chapter. Michael was driven by his need to drink. He may have acknowledged that there were other values, but he was unable to respond appropriately to them. His drinking certainly suggested a high degree of immaturity, and indicated that he was controlled by his impulses.

2. *The ability to objectify oneself: i.e., to see oneself as others do.*
Maturity helps a person, as it were, "to sit on the sideline" and look at his or her own life as an outside observer. This requires the ability to be reflective and insightful concerning one's own life without getting caught in one's own little circle. At times this vision includes glimpses of one's place or role in the much wider, even universal, perspective in which one participates as a human being. Among other qualities reflective of this level or maturity is the ability to laugh at oneself.

In a very serious way we saw this ability in Joe who, despite his grief over his wife's tragic death in a car accident, could stand back and see the demands that his responsibilities as a parent made on him, and fulfill them without being insensitive about Mary's death. To take one-self too seriously or to be too preoccupied with one's own condition is often a sign of immaturity.

3. *The ability to be guided by a unifying philosophy of life.*

Although a unifying philosophy of life is not necessarily religious in nature, it is very closely related to religious values. It indicates a direction in life that gives meaning to one's striving and activities. Religious values have the power to draw a human life together and ease it into a specific direction.

The structure of the personality provides the forum in which virtues express themselves in daily life. The virtue of faith, for instance, is expressed very differently in a fearful, insecure person than in a free and self-accepting individual. The fearful person is inclined to see God as punitive and vengeful; the free and self-accepting person experiences God as a loving parent and friend. Daily life and behavior tend to be lived according to these tendencies either in fear or in freedom. When a fearful or insecure person experiences signs of God's goodness, he or she may also develop a deeper understanding of God.

Changing one's view of God can have a freeing influence on the whole personality. James, the heavy-equipment operator injured in a construction accident, is an example of this growth and change. Slowly his need to produce made room for a more secure personal value. As this occurred his anger with God changed to confidence. Not only was the shape of his religious values related to the structure of his personality, but his religious values contributed to the growth and development of his personality structure as they were expressed.

A unifying philosophy of life and one's personality structure are extremely closely related. The healthier (i.e., the more balanced) a personality is, the more mature (i.e., the more responsible) the reaction is to the circumstances of life. A more mature individual can integrate pain and suffering into life more effectively than an immature person.

The Consequences of Illness

After recognizing the connection between suffering and maturity, it is easier to understand how certain consequences of illness can have a positive influence on human life and personal development.[2] They have the potential to deepen it or give it a new direction. There are three major and immediate consequences of illness on one's level of maturity.

1. *Illness calls forth and deepens interhuman concerns.* The patient experiences a dependence on others, whether the other be a spouse, a relative, a colleague, or a physician. The patient is forced to acknowledge his or her own limitations and will learn (sometimes reluctantly) to respect the caregiver. The condition of the patient invites the caregiver to develop gentleness, understanding, and patience according to the patient's need.

The call to take care of another person can create in the caregiver a deeper sense of personal value and importance as happened in the attitudes of Sue and her daughter after James lost his arm. In the loving caregiver this is not a sense of power or control, but rather a tendency to offer one's talents for the healing and wholeness of the patient. If, then, both patient and caregiver can see through the symbolism of life and recognize that the interaction of giving and receiving is God's creative reaching out translated into human activity, this relationship receives new depth. This depth can surpass psychological structures and give a dimension to the human reality that is simultaneously unifying and spiritual.

Illness is not only an opportunity for a deeper and more active interhuman concern, it also opens the way for the experience of dependence and confidence. The experience of human limitations emphasizes the need for dependence as a reality of human life and as a condition that is inseparably connected with being human. When care is given in a loving way, the experience of receiving care creates a sense of value in the receiver. In receiving such care a person can experience being accepted as a person with intrinsic inner value, rather than being valued solely for one's productivity or other marketable values. Receiving this type of loving care counterbalances the seemingly negative connotations of dependence and confirms a perspective and value that are easily overlooked in successful human activity.

2. Suffering calls for sharing in the work of redemption.

Human experience always involves a certain degree of imbalance between the physical, psychological, or spiritual dimensions of existence. Redemption is the restoration of the proper balance among these three dimensions of human life. Through redemption, humanity is able to respond to God's call with full human consent by allowing spiritual values to occupy a central place in the human reality, and by acknowledging God's call to humankind to live the infinite presence of the divine in created dimensions. Faith in God's presence is recognized in the acceptance of dependence.

God's central place in human life also includes confidence in God's goodness and faithfulness. God does not merely place humankind in the position of dependence as if it were a sign of lesser dignity. The dependence on God is a sharing in God's life. It is a form of interdependence in that through God's gift we are able to reach out constructively to others. Through our response, God's love is translated into created visibility. The conscious experience (acceptance) of dependence is an acknowledgement that our origin lies in God. The experience of love and care is an invitation to total surrender to the divine.

The trust we place in other people translates our confidence in God into the language of human behavior. The acceptance of care during times of illness expresses the human language of hope. It assists the patient to respond to life in the best way possible, and to make of life what it is called to be at that moment.

When we discussed the case of Edward, the young man on the respirator, we focused on his parents and his siblings (see page 89). Focusing on Edward we see a lively young man, full of fun and activity. His illness initially threw him totally off balance, but quickly he developed a remarkable ability to accept his condition. It was a joy to visit with him. He could not speak because the respirator was connected to his windpipe, but he could mouth words. While visiting with him one could talk with him (provided one could lip-read), joke with him, and also pray with him. He was not overly religious, but he accepted the fact that he was incurably ill, and that he could serve God only by being the best patient he could be. The acceptance of his condition made him more human and rooted his hope and confidence more deeply in God.

The interaction between dependence and caring creates a bond between giver and receiver. Receiving as well as giving are needs in the human person. Although they can be manifestations of "neediness" in a negative (self-seeking) sense and signs of immaturity, they can also be expressions of an inner richness that finds fullness and fulfillment in reaching out or in accepting.

Caring interaction is an active expression that mirrors God's reaching out to us and accepting our response. This caring interaction creates a bond of love that offers the opportunity for the development of the human qualities that lead to the integration of the divine presence into human life. This interaction is actually a participation in Jesus's redemptive activity.

3. Suffering leads to interhuman solidarity.
Life always searches for a higher degree of livability. This search has an individual basis, but includes a relationship with others. This relationship often creates a tension that must be solved. Peter Kreeft quoting C.S. Lewis says:

> For the wise men of old, the cardinal problem of human life was how to *conform* the soul to objective reality, and the solution was wisdom, self-discipline and virtue. For the modern mind, the cardinal problem is how to *subdue* reality to the wishes of man, and the solution is technique.[3] (Emphasis added)

The solution to the tension between conformity and control is an indispensable condition for living. It is impossible to live without tension, but tension is always a form of suffering. Greshake states this very accurately when he writes:

> People who have never endured distress have never lived. Those who are covered with wounds now healed have a special warmth. They have learned that wounds are an examination or test of life to probe our strength, our innermost convictions, our personal character.[4]

People who understand the meaning of life take their call to personal growth seriously. For them suffering becomes a comrade in arms, since the solution of the inner tension cannot be achieved without pain. Pain is never sought for its own sake but can be accepted as an indispensable companion and tool to achieve personal wholeness. Mature self-giving involves the pain of uncertainty and separation as well as the satisfaction of new growth. To run away from or to protect oneself too much from the pain of self-giving and separation is to stunt one's personal growth. Whenever personal growth is restrained, society is bound to suffer with, and because of, the individual. Dorothy Söelle explains this when she writes:

> One wonders what will become of a society in which certain forms of suffering are avoided gratuitously...in which a marriage that is perceived as unbearable quickly and smoothly ends in divorce; after divorce no scars remain. Relationships between generations are resolved as quickly as possible, without a struggle, without a trace. Periods of mourning are "sensibly" short. With haste the handicapped and the sick are removed from the house and the dead from the mind. If changing marriage partners happens as readily as trading in an old car for a new one, then the experience that one had in the unsuccessful relationship remains unproductive. From suffering nothing is learned and nothing is to be learned.[5]

Söelle does not glorify suffering for its own sake, nor does she advocate that one should never withdraw from difficult situations. She presents suffering as an unavoidable and indispensable condition that contributes to the growth of the individual and the development of others in the human community. Suffering is more than merely a social value. If we accept the spiritual dimension as an integral perspective of human wholeness, then suffering has a spiritual value.

The Rewards of Suffering

It is easy (if not simplistic), but incomplete, to say that God rewards us for the suffering that we endure. Undoubtedly, God rewards us when we accept suffering with courage and patience, but this reward is not something that we have earned or that comes to us from outside ourselves. It is a growth process that happens within the personality. This quality of self-giving can be a manifestation of the virtue of generosity. It can be described as the "availability of one's total self for the good of others without fear of loss of self."[6]

The religious perspective animates and fills this human tendency and allows the human vocation of "being the image of the creator" to be expressed in a concrete human reality and relationship. The human ability for self-realization is God's gift; the human effort to become what one is called to be is a power which also is God's gift. The activation of this power is the concurrence of the human effort and God's continuous active involvement with the individual.

Whenever suffering demands generosity in self-giving, the person's conscious spiritual perspective becomes a source of integration and wholeness. It sparks a process in which patients cease to reflect on what they could be or should be, and focus on the reality of their actual condition. They then must decide to work with that reality in the most effective way possible under the present circumstances of their illness and suffering.

In the sixth developmental stage (Intimacy vs. Isolation) we see the ability to love as a basic form of self-giving expressing itself in an openness to share. This willingness to share offers, in turn, the form in which generosity can be expressed. When these elements blend together, we can come to a sense of self-realization that is fully human. Thus human generosity, seen as an availability for self-giving, reaches beyond perceptible boundaries to form a wholeness that embraces the three-dimensional reality (physical, psychological, and spiritual) of human existence.

Adult development does not stop at the level of Intimacy vs. Isolation. It continues to the seventh stage of Generativity vs. Stagnation. This is the stage in which the self-giving of the previous stage must bear fruit. This stage searches for adequacy in interhuman relationships, for self-expression that is sufficiently assertive without being domineering, and for a relationship that can simultaneously respect one's own inner self as well as the individuality of others. This balance demands a strength that permeates every aspect of one's personality. Persistence in the search for this balance and its degree of success depend on the motivation or the philosophy of life that inspires the individual. This is also the point at which religious values enter into the person's efforts. The virtue of fortitude enables the human self to blend with the invisible yet real dimension of human wholeness.

This form of human integration is exceedingly important at times of serious illness which demand a reassessment of the value of one's personality and of one's life. It rocks the individual out of any form of complacency. Nothing can be taken for granted.

James took his health, his home, and his family for granted as long as he could effectively handle his heavy road-building machinery. The accident that took away his right arm shook him to the depths of his being. His life had to be rebuilt. His physical abilities had changed. His psychological perspective on life was no longer adequate. According to his previous standards, the value of his life had become very uncertain. He was totally absorbed in his own misfortune. He had to break out of this self-absorption in order to generate new and effective interhuman relationships. He had to reassert himself in new ways and venture onto unknown paths with different expressions of professionalism. He needed to infuse new life into his motivations for living and relating. Such a change could not be achieved in a few days. James needed a creative perseverance to build himself up and to be able once again to contribute to his family and to society.

Religious values play a significant role in a renewed pattern of motivation. James and his family had prayed often and hard, and while praying, James waited for the Lord to step in and take over. But the Lord does not do such things. God has too much respect for the great gifts of human freedom, human ability, and human self-realization. In such circumstances the religious values and the human (physical and psychological) abilities must merge and form one principle of operation. When that happened for James, a new wholeness was achieved, different from the earlier expression, but healthier and more complete despite the loss of his arm.

This stage of Generativity vs. Stagnation flows into the next stage of Integrity vs. Despair/Disgust. In this eighth and final stage of maturity, all the pieces of the mosaic of life must fall into place. At this stage the individual has developed a certain degree of balance between the various aspects of life. The person is capable of meeting the normal situations of life with adequate efficiency and can adapt where necessary without losing self-respect. Life is stable and has a somewhat predictable direction.

The individual displays a self-determination which is genuine and personal, without over-reliance on external directives and commandments. The person has the ability to assess and evaluate individual circumstances and act accordingly for personal and communal benefit and growth. This ability can be likened to the virtue of prudence, which is the ability to grasp the wholeness of a situation and act constructively in response to it.

Prudence is very important in cases of illness when all routine is broken, and most customary activities are replaced with unfamiliar happenings. Life looks different, sounds different, and must be lived differently. Such adaptations demand a calm self-assurance, an open mind for new demands, and a prudent insight to integrate the current situation into the mainstream of life. Motivation plays an important part in this process. When human motivation is filled with religious values, there is strength for integrative bonding that cannot be achieved by psychological activity alone. While many instances in life can call for this form of prudence, it has a special value in the acceptance of illness and suffering. In a special way it enables people to grow through suffering and pain.

Notes

1. Allport, *The Individual and His Religion*, p. 53.
2. van der Poel, *Theology of Health Care Ministry and the Meaning of Human Suffering*, pp. 112-14.
3. Peter Kreeft, *Making Sense Out of Suffering* (Ann Arbor, MI: Servant Books, 1986), p. 168.
4. Greshake, "Human Suffering and the Question of God," p. 40.
5. Dorothy Söelle, *Suffering* (Philadelphia: Fortress Press, 1975), p. 38.
6. van der Poel, *The Integration of Human Values*, p. 102.

Living with
the Mystery of Suffering

Throughout this book the various stages of human development with their corresponding psychological, emotional, and religious modalities have been neatly organized for greater clarity. In daily life, of course, they never appear that clear or neatly organized. While the purpose of this description has been to facilitate clearer insight, it also asks for a constant vision of the totality of human life and the complicated wholeness that is characteristic of "the fullness of being human."

Nevertheless, the role of suffering in the process of human development remains a mystery that escapes full comprehension. This role (and mystery) is rooted in the seemingly contradictory tendencies of human life to express itself as completely as possible in a material existence, and to give concrete visibility and shape to the spiritual reality of God's creative and redemptive presence. This tension is an inseparable part of the human reality and expresses itself in the personality of each individual.

Achieving Wholeness through Suffering and Pain

Without the perspective of a wholeness which integrates the physical, psychological, and spiritual dimensions into a oneness of being, suffering cannot make sense. Without a perspective that goes beyond the reaches of material existence and human knowledge, suffering will be destructive and demeaning, and unworthy of human life. Only in the perspective of a value beyond the perceptible can the inexplicable reality of pain and suffering that exists in human life become meaningful. When suffering becomes meaningful, it will also become a valuable contribution to the human process of growth and wholeness.

The following points clarify the process of the integration of suffering into daily life, and explain how people can enter into suffering knowingly, work with it more effectively, and achieve an appropriate form of wholeness.

1. *Suffering leads to the recognition of a power beyond one's control.*

Pain, illness, or other kinds of suffering usually come to us against our will and without our efforts. They are, however, undeniable realities that make us experience our limitations. They challenge the strength of our self-image, our independence, and our ability to reach out to others. Every form of suffering becomes a test case as well as an opportunity for the integration of the religious values of faith, hope, and love into everyday life.

2. *The suffering person must take a personal stand with regard to this power beyond human control.*

The nature of a person's decision is expressed in actions that will be either wholesome and integrative, or disruptive and disintegrative. The experience of suffering can be either a growth process that incorporates the physical, psychological, and spiritual dimensions of the person into a oneness, or it can cause stagnation and stunt growth and development. Accordingly, it will contribute to, or stand in the way of, spiritual growth and wholeness.

3. *Suffering leads to a realistic self-concept.*

The experience of one's limitations and the recognition of one's strengths and weaknesses are invaluable aspects of self-understanding. They pave the way to healthy and wholesome responses to all of life's challenges. Generosity, strength, and prudence on psychological as well as spiritual levels are called to unfold and flourish in the suffering person.

4. *People who suffer often discover and develop hidden talents.*

Adjustment to new conditions calls for the activation of dormant potential in the effort to engage one's total self in particular circumstances. The well-known art of mouth-painting practiced by people who have lost the use of their hands and arms is only one example of such a special development. Suffering can lead people to a new and unsuspected richness of personality. I can never forget the gentleman who was born without arms, but who grew up to be a minister and who was very active in the cause of the handicapped. His "foot-writing" was considerably better than my handwriting.

5. *Joy and satisfaction are often a result of such new developments and successes.*

A new self can be discovered which overshadows the pains of earlier disappointments. New responses create new relationships with people and with God. Suffering teaches honesty with self and with others. Meister Eckhart states accurately: "Suffering is a fast-footed animal that can carry us in the shortest possible time to the greatest possible perfection."[1]

The Example of Jesus

I consider it unforgivably irreverent and pretentious to try to psychoanalyze Jesus. Yet as the God-made-human for our sake, Jesus bears all our infirmities and shares with us the richness of his divinity. Scripture states that Jesus learned obedience through suffering (Heb 2:8–9). The total union between Jesus and God deepened and grew through the experience of suffering.

Being human like us, Jesus experienced the entire process of human and personal integration, including the slow and cumbersome path of human development. While the scriptures do not give many details about Jesus' childhood and adolescent years, we may assume that they were normal (see Lk 2:52). The years of his ministry, however, were marked by physical discomfort, and emotional and religious contradiction and adversity. We read about the discomfort of fatigue, hunger, and thirst. The gospels allow us to live through the personal pain of Jesus' rejection and ridicule by the religious leaders of his time, and the anguish of seeing his mission end as a failure (when judged by human standards). Suffering took a central place in this process.

When we reflect on Jesus' response to suffering, we see a marked difference between the earlier and the later stages of his ministry. His attitude in his early encounters with the Pharisees displayed anger but also efforts at personal integration. These conversations with scribes and pharisees were often angry encounters. This anger became violent when he witnessed the desecration of the temple. Later, however, he endured patiently their injustice and false accusations when he stood trial before Annas and Caiaphas, and then Pilate.

At the Last Supper, when he came face to face with the disciple who was about to betray him, Jesus was calm and, by any human standard, totally in control of his emotions. Dying upon the cross when he experienced the greatest possible injury and injustice, he not only remained calm and collected, but was forgiving and understanding:

"Father, forgive them, for they do not know what they do" (Lk 23:34).

By any standard of human evaluation (the only form of evaluation we can make), we see in Jesus a remarkable degree of maturation and growth. In this human growth process Jesus displayed a perfect adaptability to all the circumstances of life. We are called to achieve a similar growth in human life by adapting to circumstances and reacting according to the demands of specific moments. This process of adaptation and adjustment can only be successful if we aim at an integration that blends our human limitations with the infinite love of God.

Note

1. Meister Eckhart, as quoted by Theodore Bovet in "Human Attitudes Toward Suffering," *Humanitas*, 9.

Of Related Interest...

The Pummeled Heart
Finding Peace through Pain
Antoinette Bosco
Bosco believes that pain can be a wake-up call from God, serving to shake people out of spiritual complacency and egocentric lives.
ISBN: 0-89622-584-4, 140 pp, $7.95

Psalms for Times of Trouble
John Carmody
A realistic look at life's troubles, tempered by hope for the future based on knowledge of God's infinite love and goodness.
ISBN: 0-89622-614-X, 168 pp, $9.95

From Worry to Wellness
21 People Who Changed Their Lives
Ruth Morrison and Dawn Radtke
This book offers positive, practical ways to change for the better, as demonstrated by the stories of 21 people whom the authors have counseled.
ISBN: 0-89622-443-0, 192 pp, $7.95

Cancer and Faith
Reflections on Living with a Terminal Illness
John Carmody
This book describes how the author faced the challenge of his illness that ultimately brought him to a new understanding of faith, prayer and the fragility of human existence.
ISBN: 0-89622-594-1, 144 pp, $9.95

Available at religious bookstores or from
TWENTY-THIRD PUBLICATIONS
P.O. Box 180 • Mystic, CT 06355
1-800-321-0411

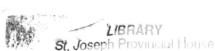